THE SALLY STRUTHERS
NATURAL BEAUTY BOOK

THE SALLY STRUTHERS NATURAL BEAUTY BOOK

Sally Struthers and Joyce Virtue
with Jane Wilkie

Illustrations by Mona Mark

Photographs by Grant Edwards

Doubleday & Company, Inc., Garden City, New York 1979

Library of Congress Cataloging in Publication Data

Struthers, Sally.
   Sally Struthers' Natural beauty book.

   Includes index.
   1. Beauty, Personal.   2. Women—Health and hygiene.
I. Virtue, Joyce, joint author.   II. Wilkie, Jane, joint author.
III. Title.   IV. Title: Natural beauty book.
RA778.S85   641.7′2
ISBN: 0-385-14350-8
Library of Congress Catalog Card Number 79-20101
Copyright © 1979 by Sally Struthers
ALL RIGHTS RESERVED
PRINTED IN THE UNITED STATES OF AMERICA
9 8 7 6 5

To my beautiful husband, B. R., and my beautiful friend, Pamela Sharp

—Sally Struthers

To my husband, Nick, and my son, Paul, for all their help, love, and encouragement

—Joyce Virtue

Contents

1. Believe Me ... 1
2. Let's Get Started ... 5
3. Skin—the Big Wrap ... 37
4. The Mane Thing ... 71
5. The Eyes Have It ... 89
6. Let's Make Up ... 97
7. What's Your Top Figure? ... 125
8. Clean Smells Good ... 153
9. Hands Up and Feet Forward ... 159
10. Voice Vibes ... 165

11. What's THAT?	*169*
12. Joyce Virtue on Vitamins and Minerals	*179*
Appendix	*191*
Meal Plan Guide for Daily Calories	*191*
Calorie Chart	*191*
Protein Chart	*197*
Food Values and Combinations	*199*
Index	*203*

THE SALLY STRUTHERS
NATURAL BEAUTY BOOK

1
Believe Me

It's odd that I should be writing a book about beauty, when I myself am not beautiful. In just the past five years, however, I've learned how to make the best of what God gave me. Which is all any of us can do.

After all, ½ per cent of women are born beautiful and stay that way. And even with perfect features, one is not necessarily beautiful. I remember seeing a TV show on which a beauty expert pointed up this fact. He showed a face totally masked, then exposed the eyes. They were lovely—large and wide set, with just the right space between eyes and brow. Then he showed the nose, also perfect. The mouth was something I've dreamed about having. Then he took the masking away completely. The face was Judy Carne, known to millions via the old "Laugh-In" show. Judy is a lovely young woman, but to my knowledge has never been renowned as a beauty.

Then he showed a second masked face. He pointed out the fault of the eyes; the distance between upper lid and eyebrow was too great. The nose, rather large. The mouth was all wrong, the lower lip much too large in contrast to the upper. The mask was removed, and there was Sophia Loren, one of the world's most beautiful women. Her features are imperfect, but put together, they add up to something wonderful. I think it's the same with Barbra Streisand—and it's great she never succumbed to having a nose job. Instead, she's made the very most of her face and because of it is unique.

It's my guess that Streisand, to many people, is a beautiful woman because she *thinks* she is beautiful. She projects the security and healthy ego of a woman who feels she's someone to look at. That's where I fail. Every time I look at Catherine Deneuve, or Sophia, my self-esteem shrinks to peanut size; I *know* I'm not beautiful, and in addition, have an awful lot of trouble making myself think I am.

Self-opinion begins at an early age, and tends to stick. From thirteen to nineteen, I wondered if it was worthwhile to live to my twentieth birthday. I felt I was dumpy. My sister called me Packy, a nickname standing for pachyderm—which means elephant, standing or otherwise.

I was convinced I was ugly, an impression compounded every time I looked at my round face in a mirror. My mom tells me I was *born* with a round face. "That round face on top of that skinny little baby's body," she says. "When you were bundled up with just your face exposed, everyone commented on what a healthy, fat baby I had." I was condemned from infancy—all my life people would think I was heavy because of the shape of my face.

I was always the shortest kid in my class. People patted me on the head and pinched my cheek a lot. You know the routine—"You cute little kid." To this day, I shudder when anyone pats me on the head (they still do), and grow rigid like a cat facing off a dog whenever anybody reaches thumb and forefinger toward my cheek. A tweaked cheek is devastating when you're an adult, so I wear platform shoes to fend off life's tweakers.

I had a "funny walk," people said, probably because I wore corrective shoes. My arches weren't forming correctly. I still have a funny walk, a gait all my own. Part of it is due to the balancing act needed with platform shoes. But I realize that my style of sallying—an action of rushing or bursting forth—also comes from my self-image. Everyone's posture and style of walking is patterned after the way they've been programmed to believe they look. Since I believed I was ugly and *knew* I was short, I walked fast to keep up with others, but with short, comical, hard steps. Always the clown.

I was very young when I noticed the deep cleft in my chin, and when I asked about it, I heard that after God makes babies He reviews them in sort of an assembly line and tweaks the cheeks of the ones He likes. (According to rumor, God, too, has that awful habit.) And with the babies He doesn't like, He puts his thumb on their chin and shoves them away. This explanation sank in like a stone, and after that, when I said my prayers, I always covered my chin with my hands to hide the cleft so maybe God would forget He hadn't liked me on Day One.

Mother Nature did try to even the score by giving me white, even teeth, but when a front tooth was knocked out when I was in the seventh grade, a dentist filled up the space with a shiny silver tooth, just as big as the late departed one. I could send secret messages to Captain Midnight when I smiled during a full moon.

When I finally got a bosom, I got one so big that I busted a lot of blouse buttons. And when you have a big bosom below a round face, there is no way people will not believe you're fat all over.

All that stuff is why I'm writing this book. I fell into a trap of believing I was a hopeless case and, most important, *funny looking.* You know what that did to me, that feeling like a munchkin all the time? It never went away, and so that funny-looking person is still inside me. No matter how hard I try to believe otherwise, that person pops out every once in a while to get the best of me. Definitely not fun.

How about you? Do you have problems you don't know how to solve? Or problems you think *can't* be solved?

Perhaps I can help. I've had my own lessons to learn, and can pass on some helpful advice. More importantly, I have Joyce Virtue as a friend. In a Beverly Hills beauty salon, Joyce gives advice on skin care and makeup to actresses like Mary Tyler Moore, Sandy Duncan, Patty Duke, and Cloris Leachman.

Joyce knew all the basics a long time ago, having been a model and a dancer, and one of the first things you learn in show business is the art of makeup. But ten years ago, Joyce had a bout with migraine headaches and vertigo, and the prescribed drugs only made her feel worse. So she began studying health and nutrition, and today is a licensed cosmetician and makeup artist, with a master's degree in Nutrition and a doctorate in Naturopathy—which is drugless therapy. Joyce fairly spouts information about things like agar (seaweed) for dry hair, oil of wintergreen for your feet, and potato compress for circles under your eyes. When Joyce says drugless, she means drugLESS. Everything she's taught me how to use are nature's own products; many are things you have in your kitchen. So while we're teaching you how to be beautiful, you'll be doing it cheaply. Corn oil and eggs, for example, are a lot less expensive than endless jars of commercially made beauty products, most of which don't improve you one bit. Furthermore, they cost you a bundle because you pay not only for the packaging, but the advertising as well. The things Joyce uses you can buy by the ounce, in paper sacks, so to speak.

In this book you're going to bump into a lot of creations new to you. All are natural products, without chemicals. They come from the earth, as we do; both the Bible and Darwin have us coming from down under.

If you ask, "What are little girls made of?" the answer is not sugar and spice. Both girls and boys are made of water, proteins, and minerals, plus about one ounce of vitamins, at the moment of birth. Minerals are as important as vitamins in the maintenance of health because the body cannot manufacture additional minerals and must rely on outside sources. The practice of Naturopathy teaches you how to replenish the body with all the things we're made of in the first place.

When Joyce first mentioned to me things like burdock root, comfrey and golden seal tea, I always said, "What's THAT?" And then, "Where do you buy it?" So, for your education in the world of nature, Chapter 11 of this book is a very small encyclopedia titled "What's THAT?." It will answer all your questions.

I first met Ms. Virtue when I went to her for a makeup job before appearing on the "Sonny and Cher Show," and when she finished with this chubby face of mine, I had never looked so good. While Joyce was working on me she talked about skin care related to general health, and I was fascinated. I'd never known anyone so knowledgeable about beauty. Joyce herself is living, vibrant proof. Having practiced what she preaches, she's in her mid-forties but looks a fast twenty-five and is absolutely gorgeous from head to toe. See picture on page 17. We've been close friends for seven years now, and in that time I've digested a lot of her know-how.

I think there are thousands of you out there with problems that distress you. So when I told Joyce I wanted to write an honest book about beauty and needed her help, she jumped in with both feet . . . which, incidentally, are also beautiful. In the case of Joyce Virtue jumping with both feet, this can amount to a considerable thud. She's no hippo, but she's crammed with knowledge and wants to include all of it. This is fine with me, but I want to assure you that there aren't enough hours in a day to do everything she recommends. So don't panic at the tremendous scope in the book. You can pick and choose for yourself—try just one natural facial, maybe only one herbal hair rinse—but I know that anything you try and practice is guaranteed to improve you in that particular area. I look at it this way . . . if you learn only one thing—how to treat sunburn or when to take your vitamins—reading my book will have been worthwhile.

While I'm working on it, Joyce is over my shoulder almost every minute, and, in fact, has contributed an entire chapter on vitamins. She is also the source for all the "hard facts" in this book and is responsible for the material in the Appendix.

There you are. I promise you that Joyce knows more about beauty and body chemistry and diet and vitamins and skin care than many doctors.

So, with her help, when I tell you something, you'd better believe it.

2
Let's Get Started

I repeat, you don't have to do *everything* I recommend—and I don't want you to feel guilty if you skip a lot of things—but if you want to get the very best results from anything you do try, you should first be in the best health possible.

I'm in that happy state these days, and doubly appreciate it because I was sick a lot when I was a kid. I had pneumonia and pleurisy and infectious mononucleosis and nephritis and a dozen or so strep throats. Fortunately, not all at the same time. It seemed every germ floating by picked on me as its nest. But after a while I realized I was almost making myself ill in order to get attention from my parents, particularly my father, who was a doctor. I stopped all that nonsense when facing the fact I wasn't having much fun being in bed all the time with a thermometer hanging out of my mouth. Hypochondria is a pathetic way of getting attention. You can make yourself sick, and you can make yourself well, if you want to. (The same applies to your appearance, which can be A+ or zilch.)

You probably aren't sick, but you're very likely not healthy, either. Maybe you're in the habit of ingesting fizzy drinks and greasy hamburgers or—the worst thing I can think of—french fries topped with catsup. This sort of intake is quickly going to turn you gray or green, blemish your skin, give you wrinkles, and maybe even make you keel over . . . the latter known in my world as The Big Thud.

Before I tell you what you should eat, I'm going to suggest you get rid of the gunk that is now inside you. Please don't take offense—all we human beings are full of toxic stuff that is murder on the system. These toxins can come from fast foods, the preservatives in many things we buy at the supermarket, or even from a well-intended piece of fruit that hasn't been properly washed.

So you go on a fast—for only three days. This does not mean you're going to starve. More people die from the results of overeating than from well-regulated fasts. I think you should first understand what fasting is; what it accomplishes. It is a rejuvenating process and does wonders for every part of your body—losing a bit of weight along the way. I assure you it will make you feel great. (Joyce even plays tennis while she's fasting.) And it's not the Mohandas Gandhi type of thing, staying empty for weeks and shriveling up.

Here's how. The first thing you do is make a batch of fasting broth, which you can drink as often as you like during the three days. After chopping, place the tops of one bunch of carrots, tops of one bunch of beets, a full stalk of celery with its leaves, and one whole potato in two quarts of boiling water. You can also add chopped zucchini if you like. Simmer for thirty minutes, strain, and you have your broth. Don't knock it until you have tried it; the flavor is surprisingly good.

During the first and second days you can also drink fresh fruit juices, mixed half with water to cut the acidity—but not at the same time as the fasting broth. Throughout the three days you can have herb tea—*any* herb tea available at health food stores. And on all three days drink lots of water, six to eight glasses. Why so much water? It flushes the system, works wonders for your circulation, and aids in digestion. When you drink a lot of water, much moisture gets beneath the surface of your skin, giving your complexion a youthful look.

On the fourth day and forever after (except for occasional fasts, which I recommend highly), you can eat solid food. *Which* foods are important; guidelines will be given throughout the book, particularly in the chapters on skin and figure, and in the Appendix.

Okay, so what does all this restraint do for you?

The digestive system rests and heals. The body lives off itself, so that much over-age tissue is reduced and there's stimulation for new growth. When living off itself, the body burns up dead cells, diseased tissue, toxic waste, and what Joyce so daintily calls "morbid matter." In brief, you're getting rid of the poisons that have been lying around in there for too long.

How do they make their exit? Through bowels, lungs, kidneys, and skin . . . more through the skin than the other three combined. (Joyce has taught me to give the whole business a bit of help by taking a laxative the evening before I begin the fast. If you do this, choose a natural laxative such as Senekot—or any herb tea containing cascara sagrada. You can buy herbal laxatives at health food stores—HFS, hereafter).

While your body is cleaning house you should be careful to shower regularly, and it's a good idea to use a loofa sponge. (See "What's THAT?"

LET'S GET STARTED 7

if you don't already know.) After all, if the majority of toxins are coming out of your pores, you ought to take extra care to keep clean.

It's possible that fasting will temporarily worsen the appearance of your skin, but I hasten to assure you it quickly improves. If you notice blemishes, apply cucumber juice to your skin, or take the juice internally. Cucumber juice is available at HFS—or you can squeeze it yourself with a fruit press.

If you make a habit of fasting a few days every three months or so and get yourself into good condition, you'll find at the end of each fast that your old skin peels off and the new one looks like a baby's skin, almost as though you'd had a face peel. It doesn't peel like sunburn—it's removed when you bathe, and the exodus is better accomplished if you use a loofa sponge. Furthermore, you might even lose a few pounds. But don't count on this as permanent weight loss unless you eat sensibly after your fast.

Incidentally, when you lose weight during a fast, you don't become wrinkled or flabby because your collagen (the cementlike protein that holds our cells together) will be strengthened, and elasticity restored. Your complexion will have new life and muscle tone, and be firmer than before.

As with any change in diet, consult your physician to ascertain if you're a likely candidate for this fast. If you do tackle it, you'll react better and faster to every beauty tip in this book.

I have one more stunner for you before getting on to easier things. If you don't smoke or drink, turn the page. If you do either, stay with me for a minute. We all know neither is good for us. Both cause serious loss of vitamins, both tend to rupture capillaries of the skin. Alcohol causes a red and mottled complexion. Drinking is so socially acceptable that we often lose sight of the fact alcohol is a drug, and once in the bloodstream, turns to sugar. It's also toxic. The inhalation of smoke depletes your system of vitamin C, the vitamin essential to the formation of collagen. A dearth of it causes the face to puff—and puffy faces are not what we are after.

I don't, thank God, have the disease of alcoholism, so I don't know how difficult it is to forego drinking. I did used to smoke, though, and I know all about that particular battle. I can hear you out there, screaming, thinking that if you're going to have to stop smoking before you can be gorgeous, you'll give up the whole project. Please don't give up. Try. At least, do cut down. Think about how badly you must smell to non-smokers. You bathe and spray and perfume yourself like crazy so that you won't offend others with body odor. Why do you think that tobacco breath and the odor of cigarettes in your hair and on your skin and clothing are any less offensive than B.O.? You'll get help from the regimen you'll be on, with diet and exercise, which will make you feel so much better mentally and physically that you'll have added strength to wage the battle against tar, nicotine, and alcohol.

So much for those two "monkeys-on-the-back."

The first thing to do any morning, whether or not you are fasting, smoking, or drinking (not, I hope, in the morning), is to drink a full glass of water, preferably at room temperature. This helps the elimination process.

Next, take your morning vitamins with a glass of juice diluted with water thus supplying nutrition along with the pills. Which brings us to the subject of

VITAMINS

Once you've read the list of vitamins you should take, you'll very probably react to the number of pills. I agree they're a lot to swallow, but believe me—and Joyce—they are all necessary.

Vitamins are essential because they are catalysts in the slow and steady oxidation of protein, fats, and carbohydrates into energy. Vitamins also aid in the regulation and control of all our vital processes. Their proper intake can do nothing but improve you if—and I can't make this point too strongly—they are supplemented with a nutritious diet. With or without vitamins, if you don't eat, you're in serious trouble.

My husband, Bill, is a psychiatrist and as such has a degree in medicine, so he knows what's good for me, and is nice enough to lay out my morning vitamins on the bathroom counter. I'm lucky, because not all doctors understand the importance of vitamins and good nutrition. If the pills are still there when Bill comes home from his office, I catch it. My only excuse is that I was in a tearing hurry to take off for the studio, and I get furious with myself when I forget to take them. Without fail, every day, we should have specific vitamins.

Here are those that wake you up and keep you going during the day. Every morning you should take:

1 Chelated One-A-Day with minerals and amino acids
1 Vitamin C, 500 mg.
1 B complex
1 Vitamin B_6
1 Vitamin E, 200 IU
1 RNA/DNA (twice a week)

LET'S GET STARTED

Joyce says it's important to know that if you take Premarin in the morning skip vitamin E until 12 hours later, or at bedtime. And check with your doctor if you have high blood pressure. The reason: Dr. Wilfred Shute has found through research on vitamin E that massive doses of E lead to rapid improvement in many people afflicted with hypertension or high blood pressure. But in a few patients, the blood pressure actually rose with intake of vitamin E. So check with your doctor before you take vitamin E. Also, Premarin is antagonistic to E and they nullify each other; therefore, should be taken 12 hours apart. If you are on the Pill, take folic acid once a day.

At bedtime, take the following, which work best while you sleep and the body is repairing itself.

1 Vitamin C, 500 mg.
1 B complex
2 Calcium lactate tablets
1 Vitamins A and D, combined

Joyce warns that calcium dosage shouldn't exceed 1,200 mg. daily. So count milligrams in your One-A-Day and the chelated mineral, then check the strength of your calcium tablets so you're aware of your daily calcium dosage.

I used to bruise easily and badly. If I bumped into anything, even gently, I'd get an enormous bruise that lasted for weeks. My doctor said the reason was my deficiency of calcium and vitamin C. That was before I knew Joyce, who has taught me about vitamins and wants to explain them to you . . . plus minerals and a few other items you don't *need* to know . . . but if you're curious about these things, as I was, read Chapter 12, "Joyce Virtue on Vitamins and Minerals."

EXERCISES

No breakfast yet. Exercises follow the morning water and vitamins with juice. On the first day, you'll do three.

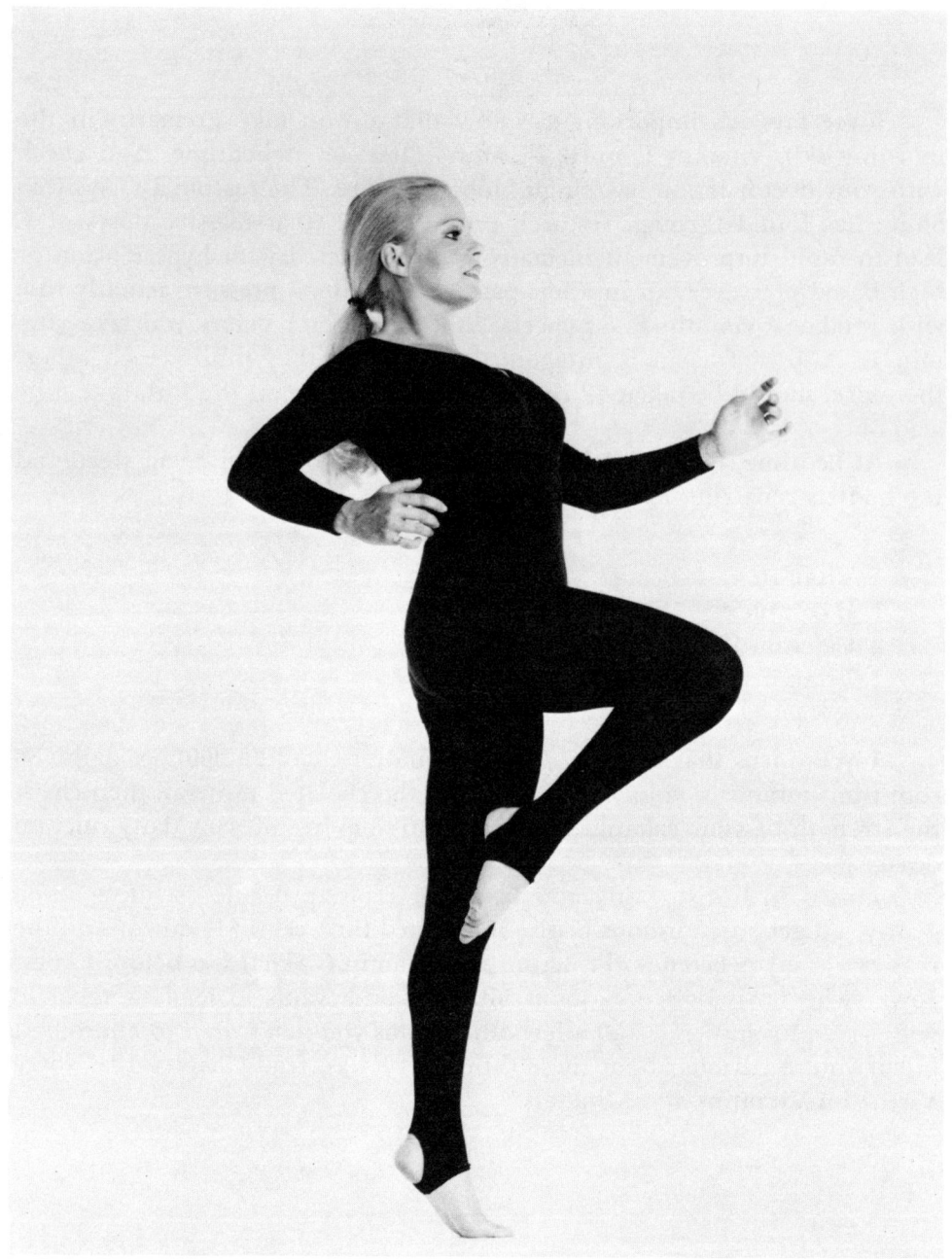

1. Jog in place for 1 minute—on a carpeted area if you have neighbors downstairs. Bend arms at your sides and hold them close to the body. Relax, don't tense. Pick up your legs as you jog, just high enough to get some movement going without straining. Do it at a comfortable pace—running is not a "comfortable" pace.

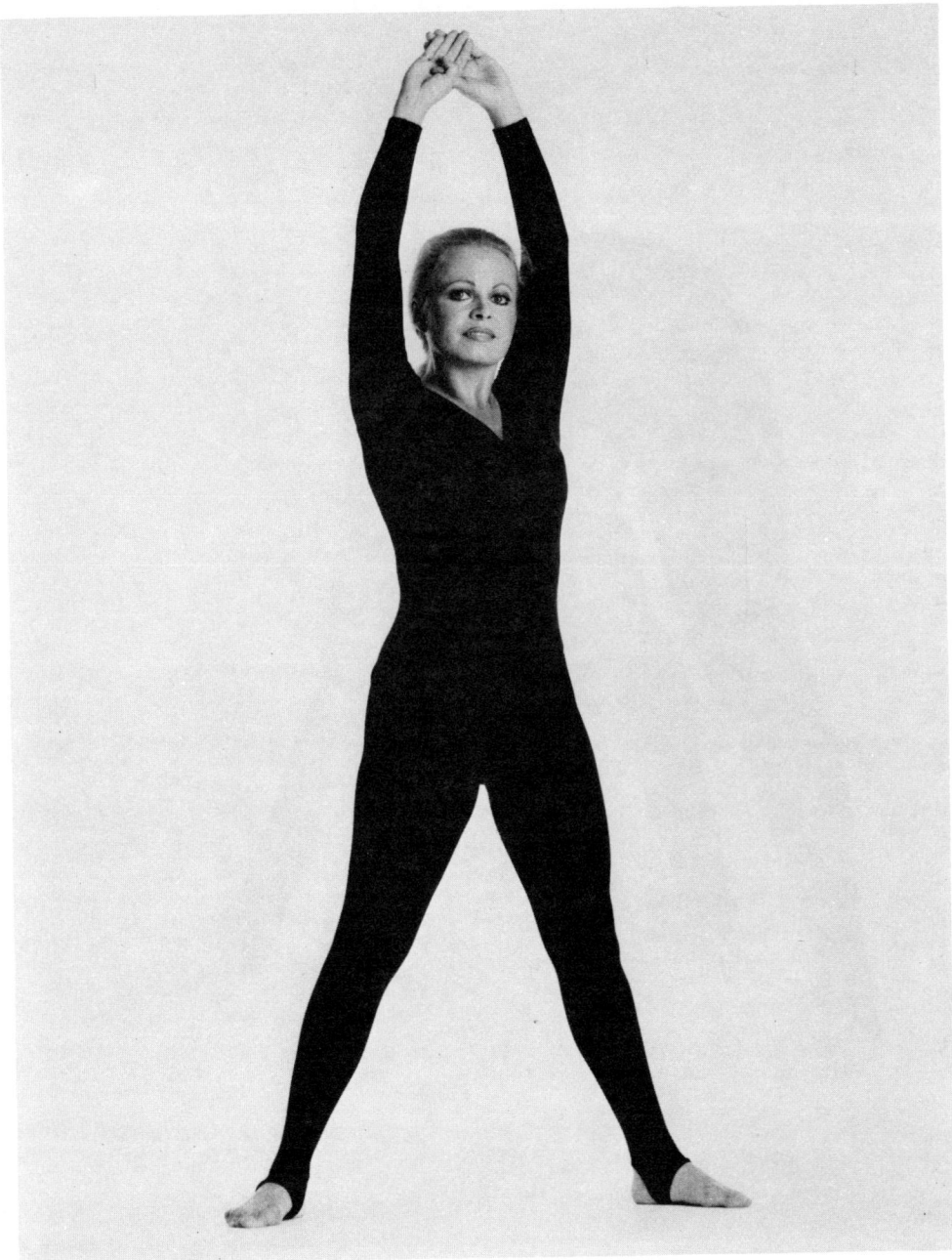

2. Stretch and pull, 10 times. Lift your arms and reach for the ceiling. In one sweep, drop the torso from the waist, keeping your head between

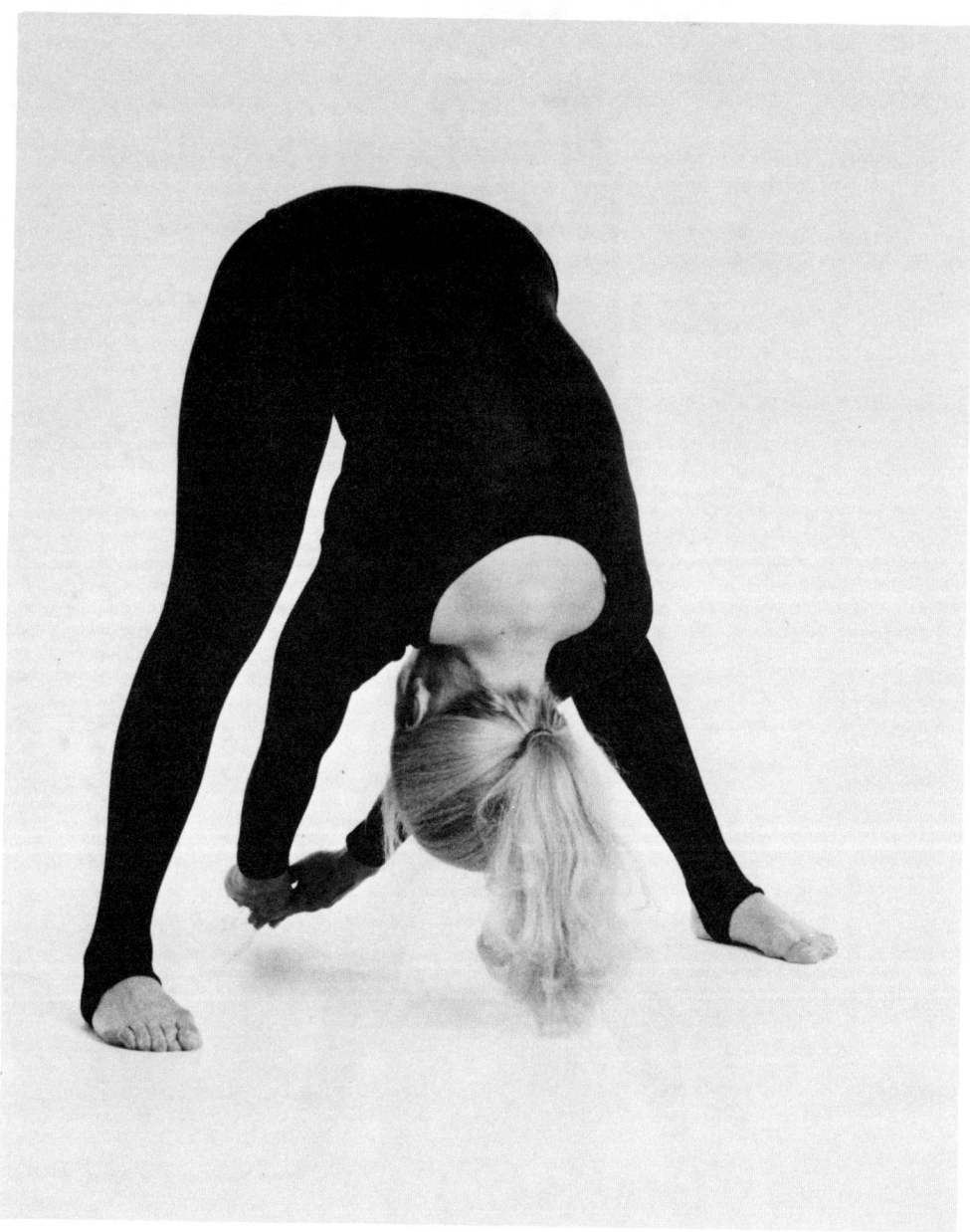

your arms, and stretch arms behind you, between your legs. Your head will be close to your knees as your arms pull back. This is an excellent exercise for blood circulation.

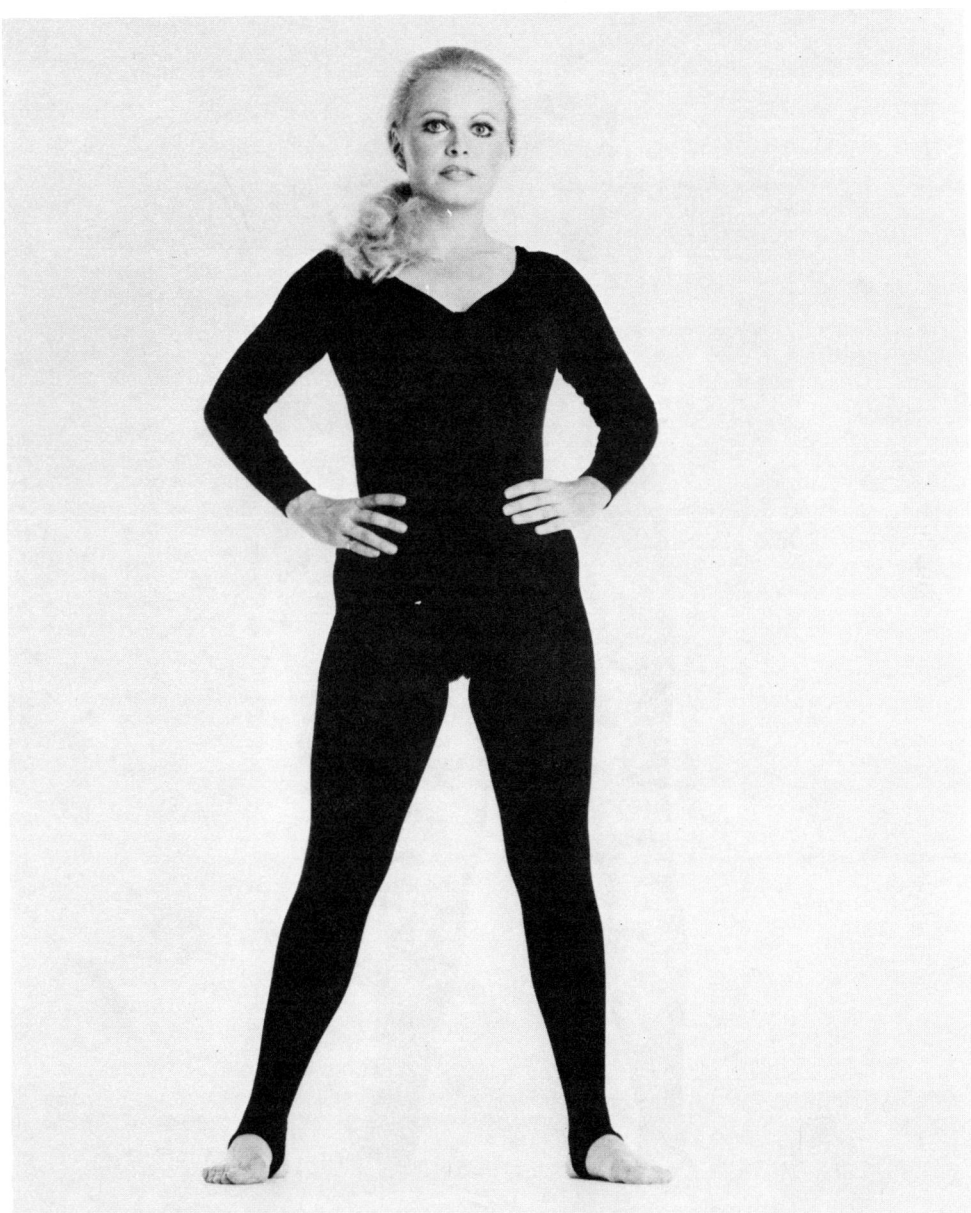

3. Side to side, stretch and pull, 10 times on each side. Straighten up, pull in your tummy and tighten your buttocks. Stretch to the left, pulling

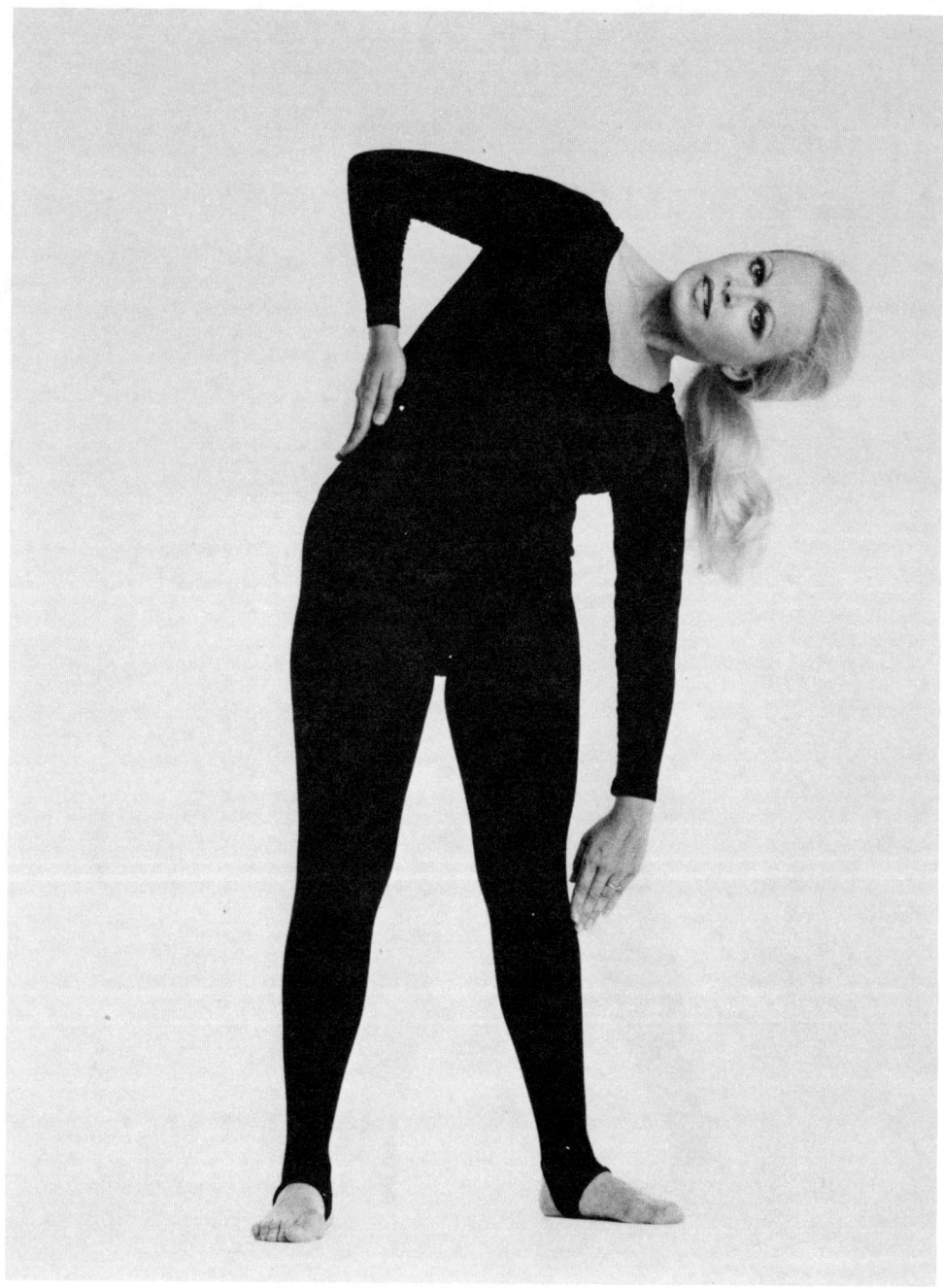

your left arm down your left leg. Stretch to the right and pull the right arm down your right leg. As you stretch and pull from side to side, move only the upper part of your torso. This is a great toning exercise and good for all parts of your body, especially the waist.

After exercising, take a warm shower and stimulate your skin with a loofa sponge. If you can stand it, finish with a spray of cold water to close your pores. This is an invigorating way to start the day.

On the second day, add three more exercises.

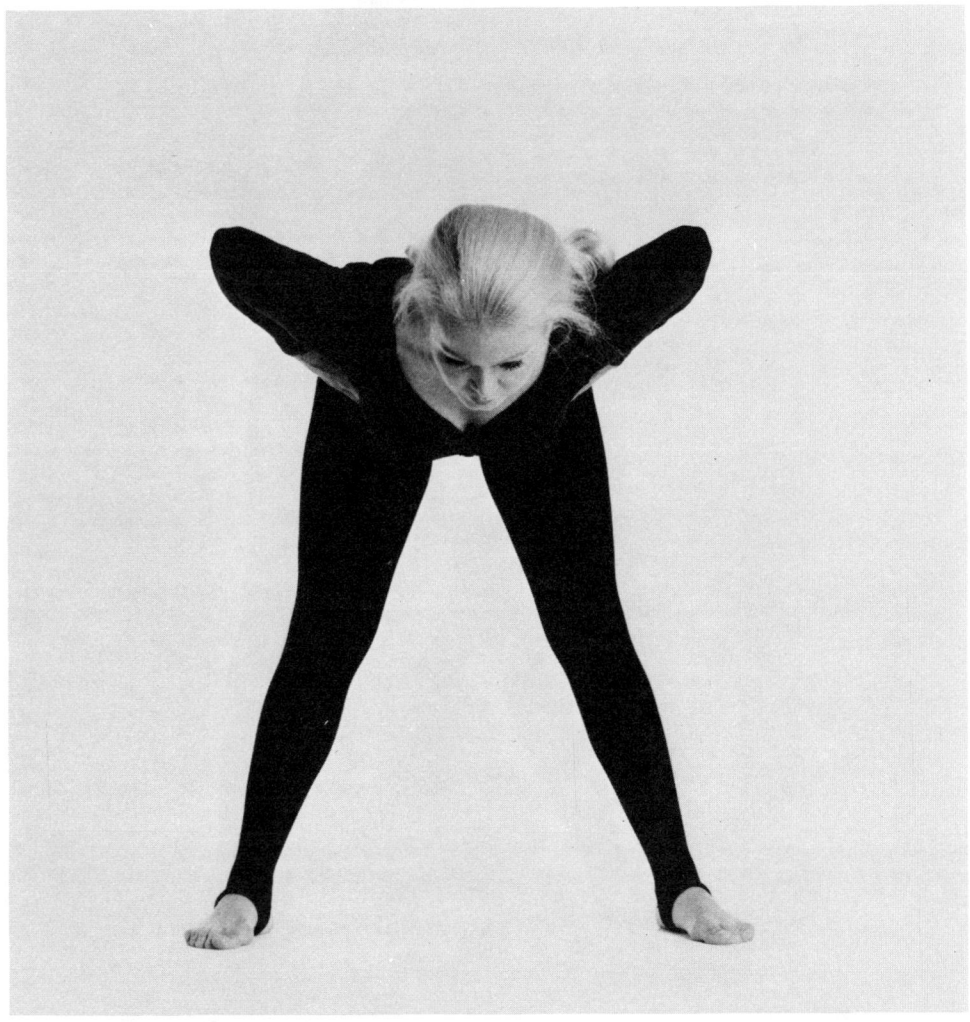

4. Make circles with your upper torso by standing with feet slightly apart and placing your hands on hips. Start by bending forward from the waist, then circle your torso around to the right as far as you can, and re-

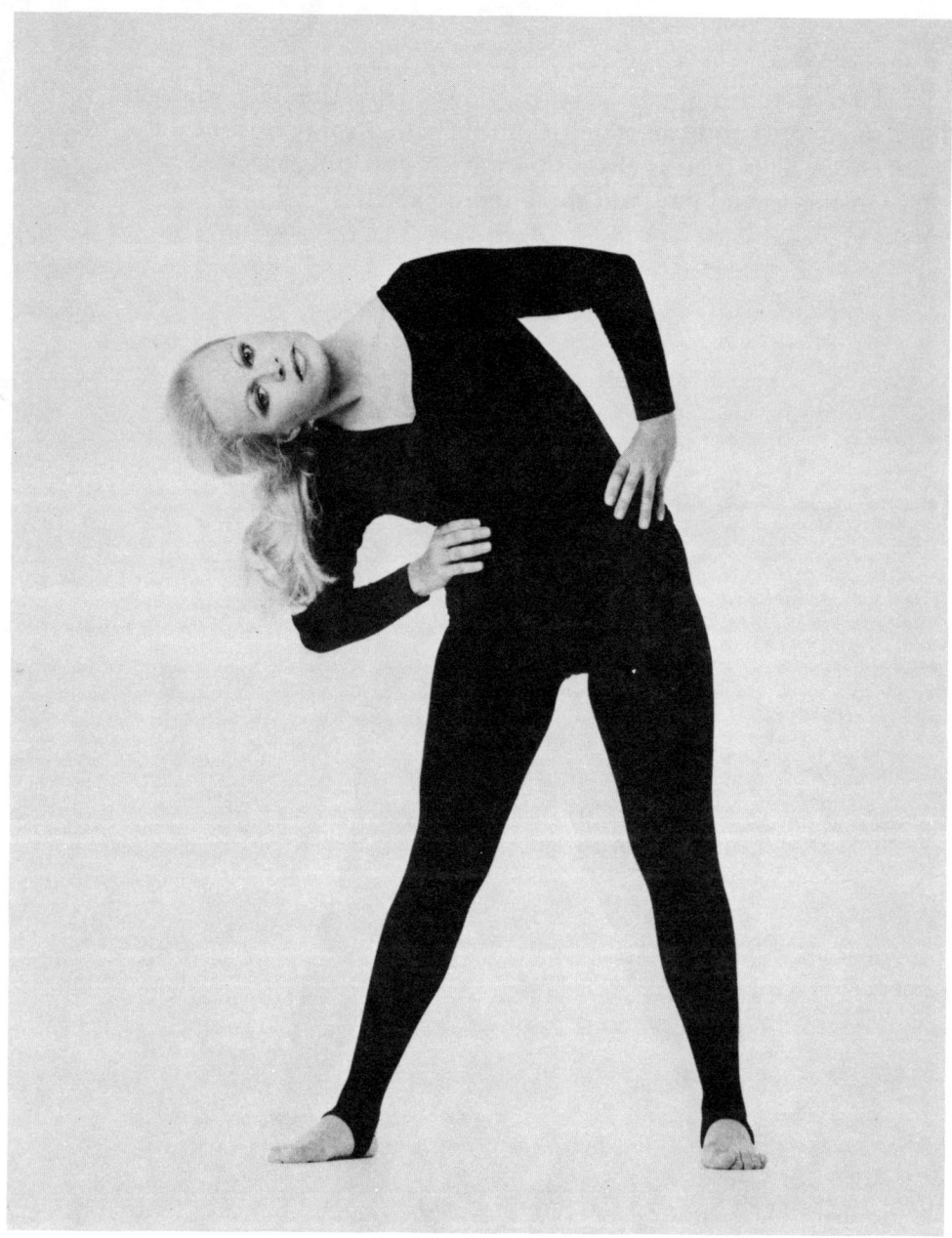

turn shoulders to normal position. Do 5 times, then 5 times to the left. This exercise is excellent for the waistline.

LET'S GET STARTED 17

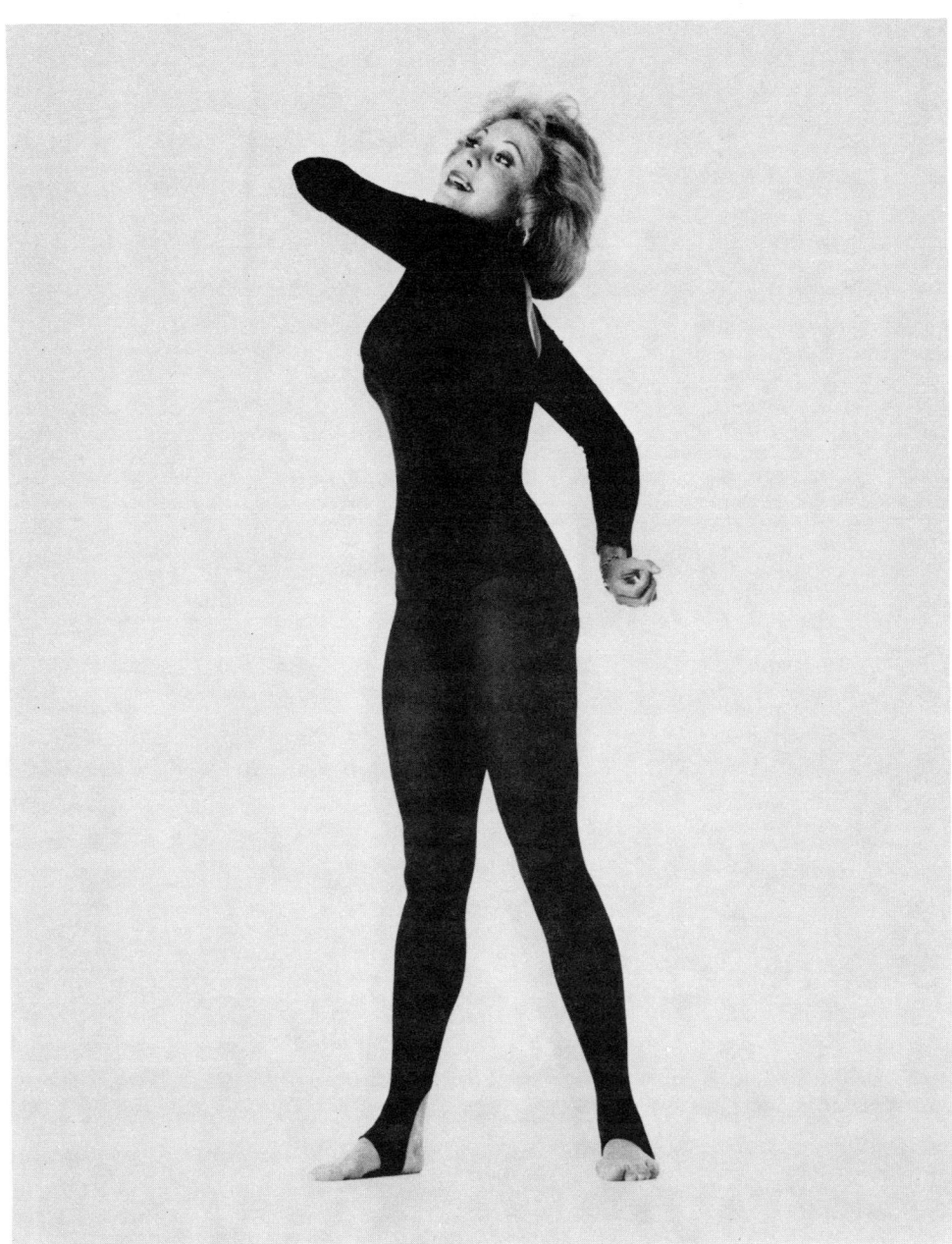

5. Another waistline special is even simpler. Stand with feet slightly apart, to help keep your balance, and twist your torso to your right, swinging arms with you as you go, then twist all the way to your left. A good way

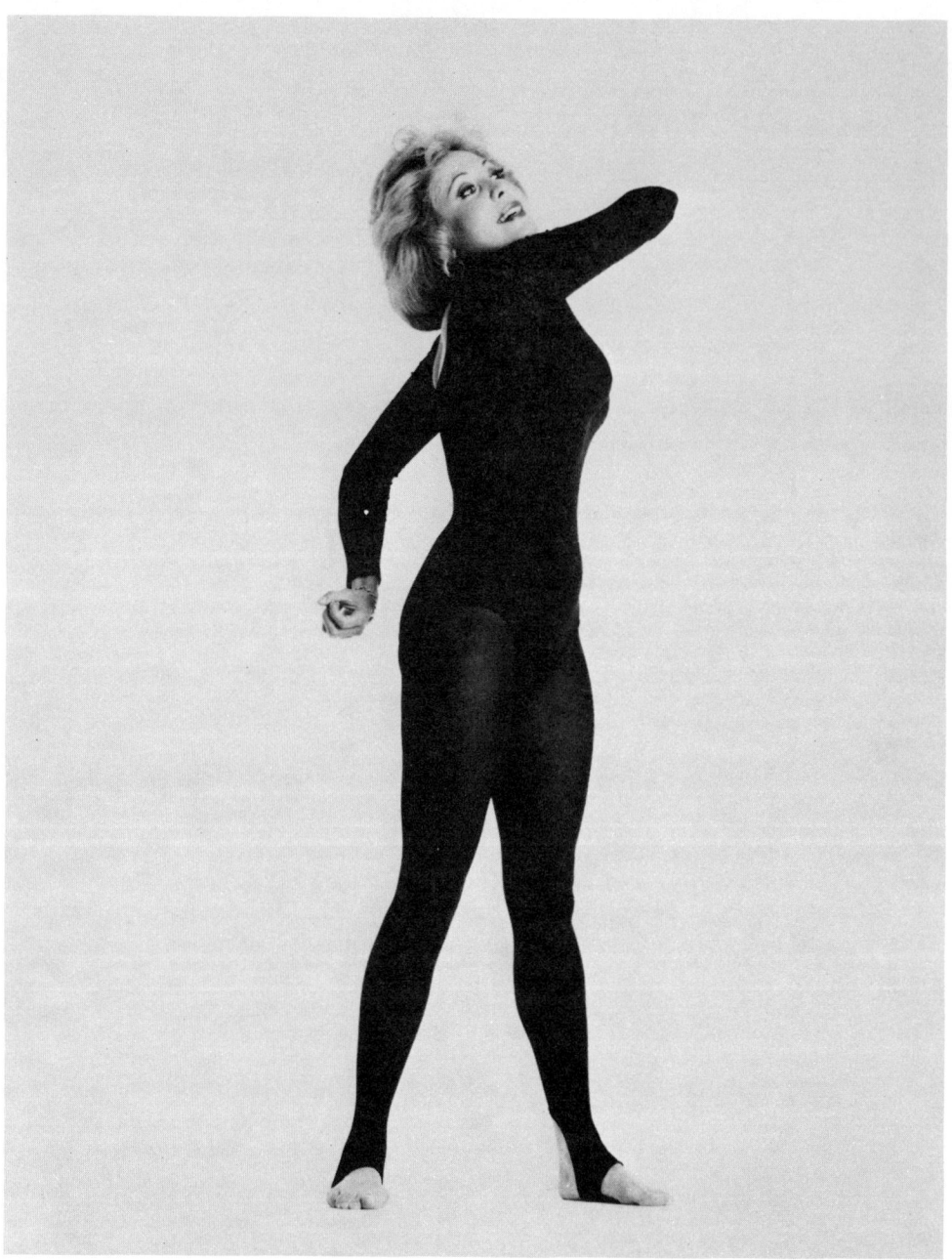

to check how well you're doing is to choose a spot on the wall behind you and try to look at it with each turn. The exercise should be done in one continuous motion until you've twisted 10 times to each side.

LET'S GET STARTED 19

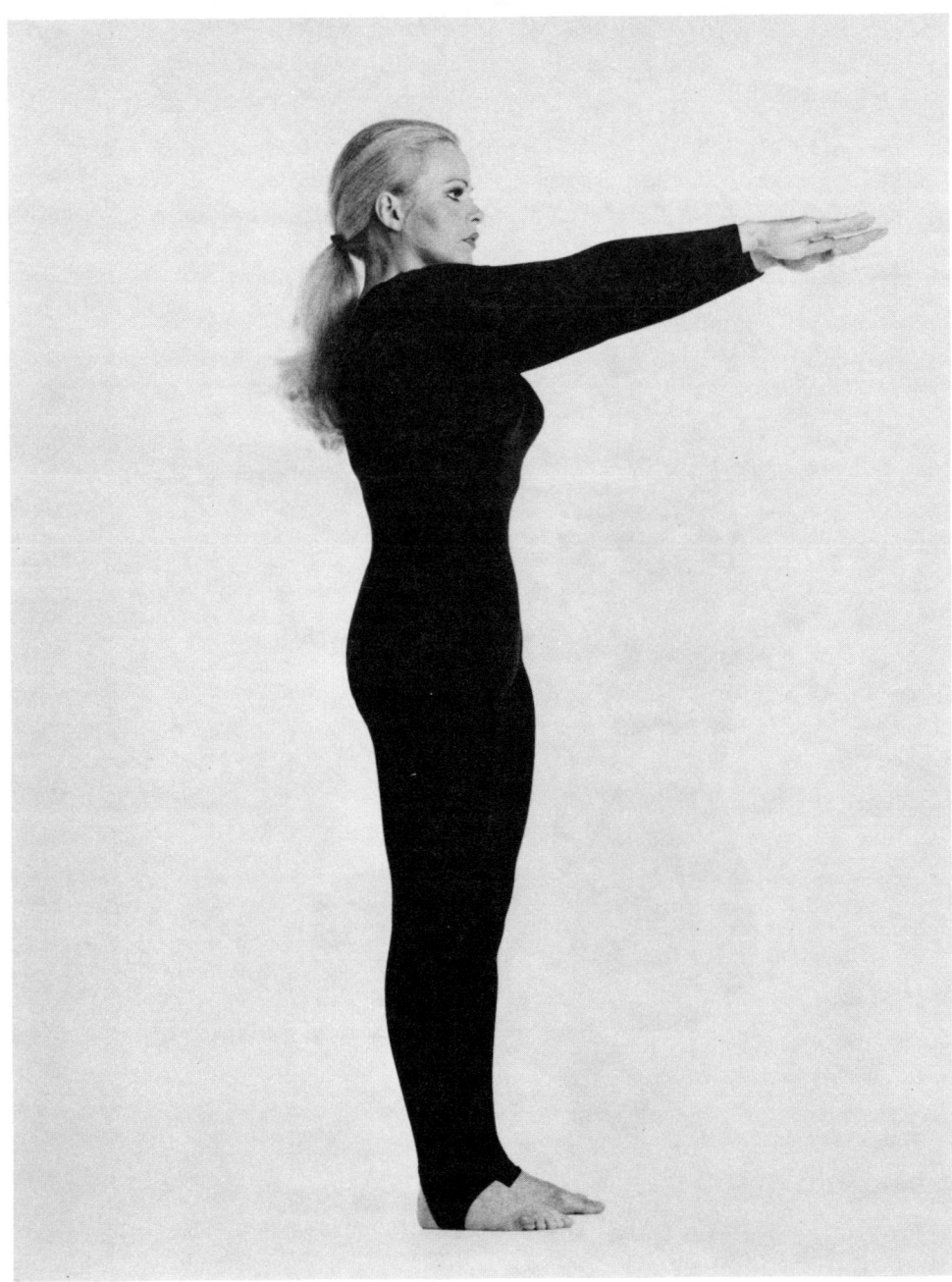

6. Knee bends are great for toning the thighs. Stand with your feet together and arms straight out in front of you. Slowly bend your knees until you're as low as possible without losing balance, then slowly stand up. You should do this without bending forward any part of your body; if

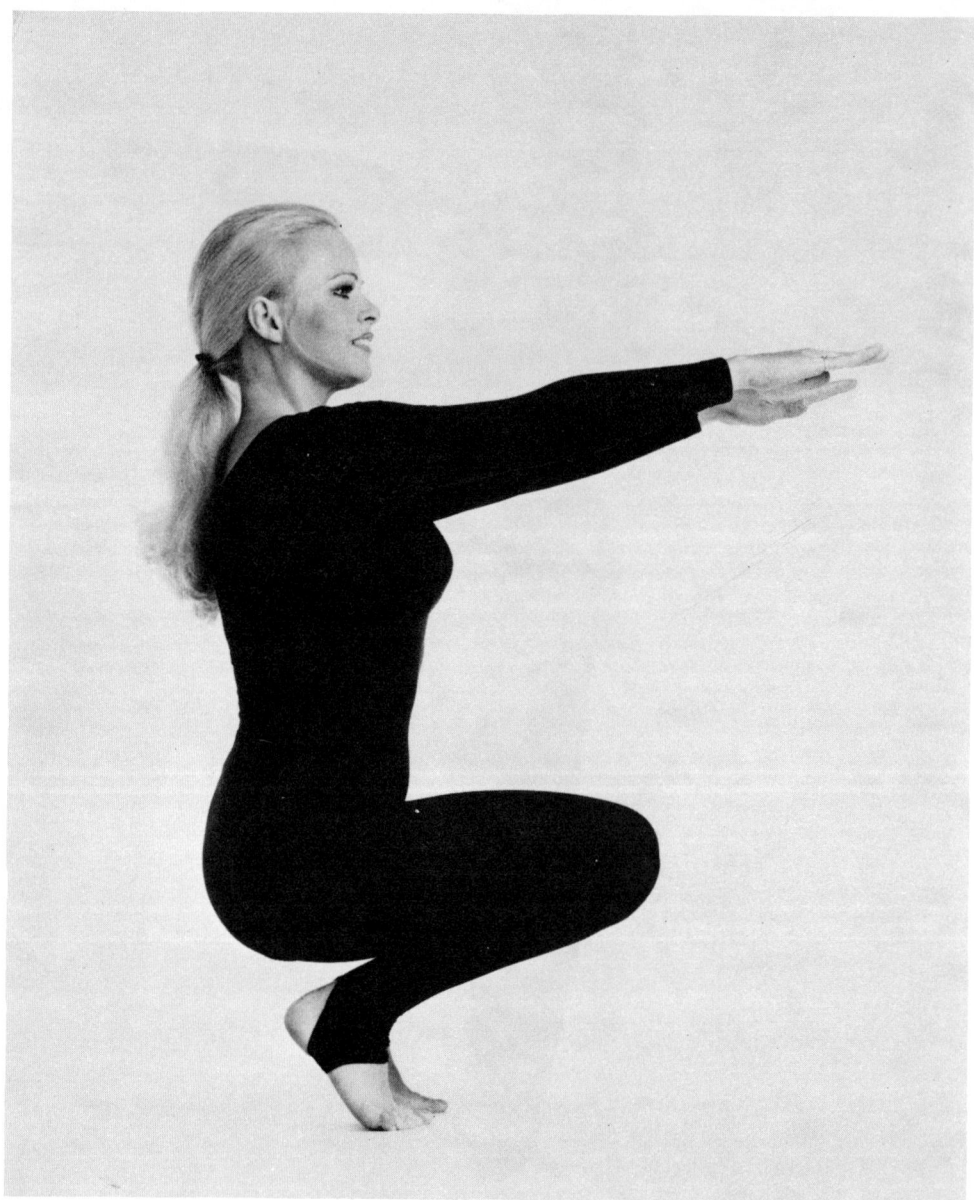

you're good enough, you can balance a book on your head to make sure your posture is erect. This really makes the thigh muscles work. Start with 3 or 4 knee bends and add one every day until you're doing between 15 and 20 daily.

LET'S GET STARTED 21

The third day.
If you're slightly winded after completing the foregoing six exercises, lie on your back and deep breathe for a few moments. Inhale through your nose, hold for a few seconds, then exhale slowly through your mouth. After three of these, you'll be breathing normally again.

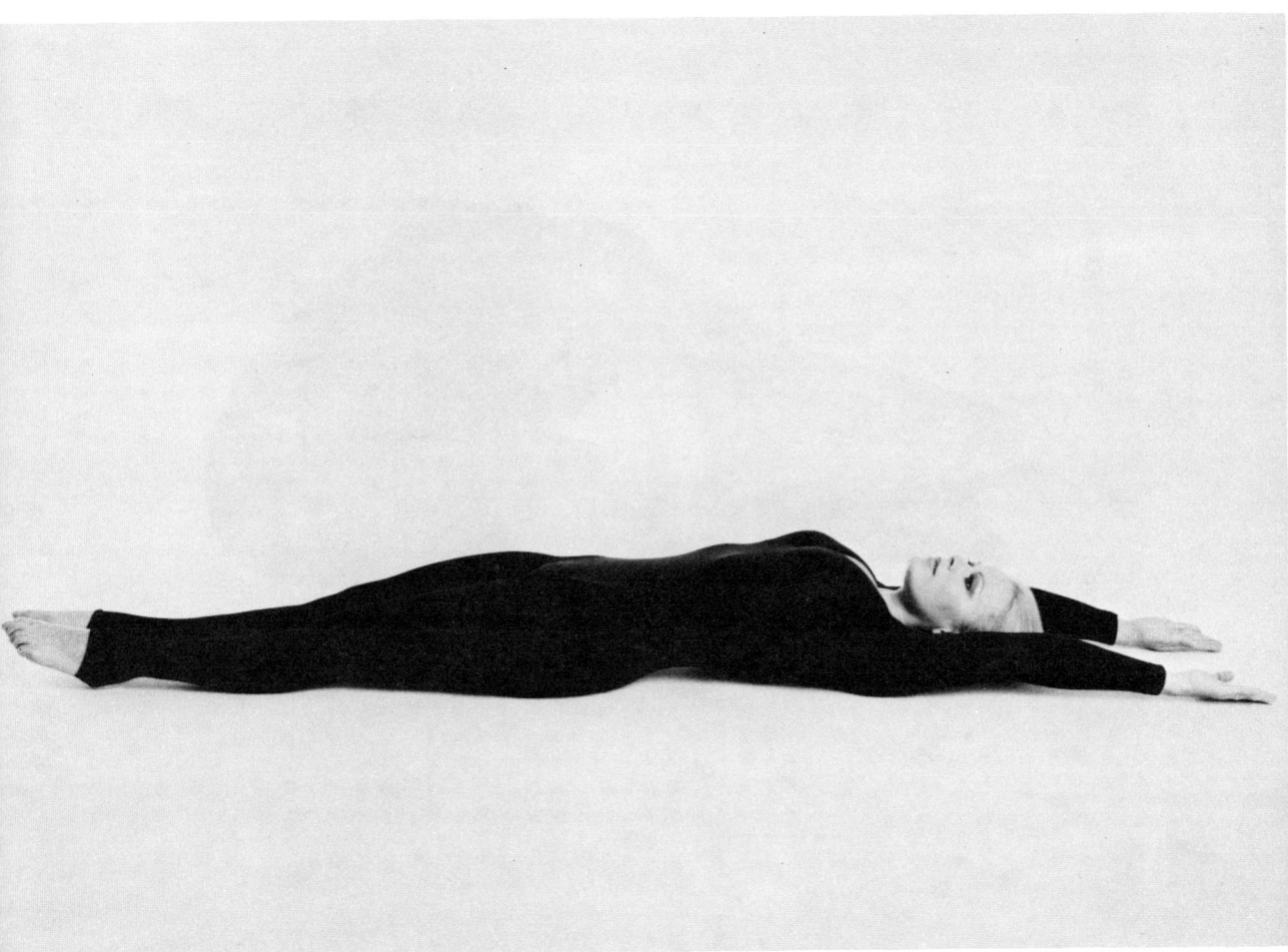

7. I got you on the floor for a purpose—the first new exercise for today is sit-ups. They are most beneficial when done with legs flat on the floor and toes pointed. Sit up, bend as far forward as possible, trying to touch

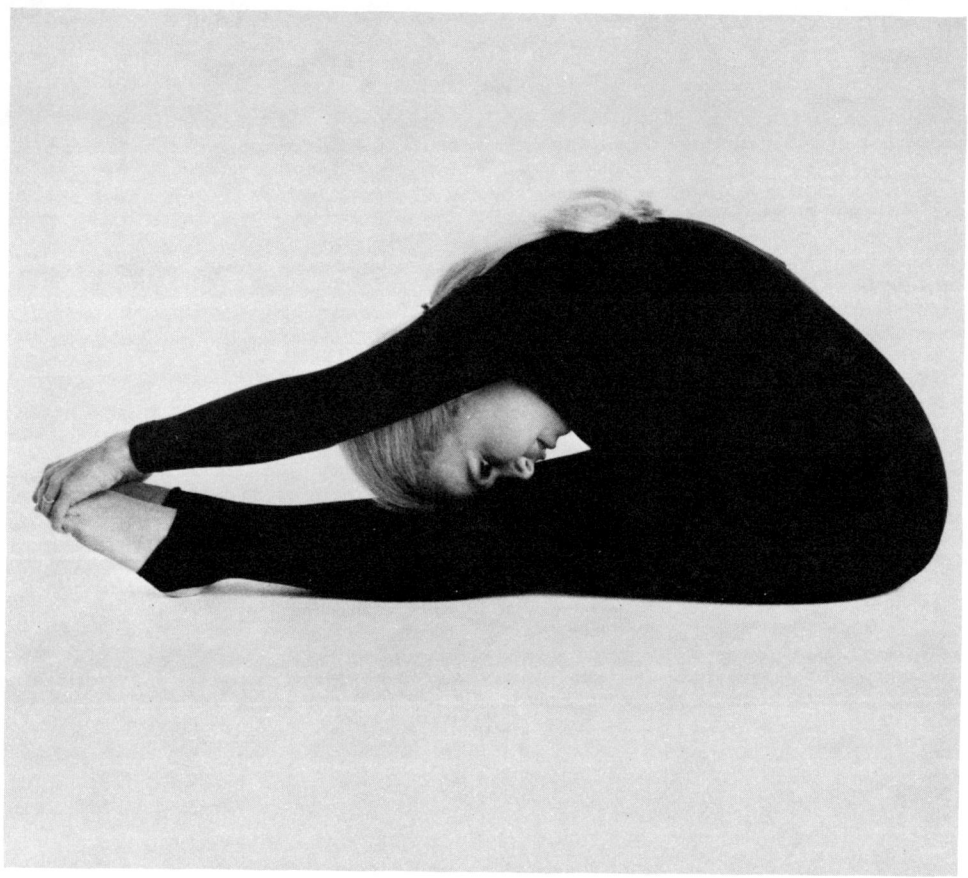

your toes, then slowly lower yourself back to the floor, with arms straight out behind you. Today, 5 is plenty to start with, then add one each day until you're up to 15 or 20. I must note here that if you have any back problems, it's best to do the sit-ups with your legs slightly bent . . . bend your knees with your feet flat on the floor, then do the sit-ups as instructed. Your back will thank you.

LET'S GET STARTED 23

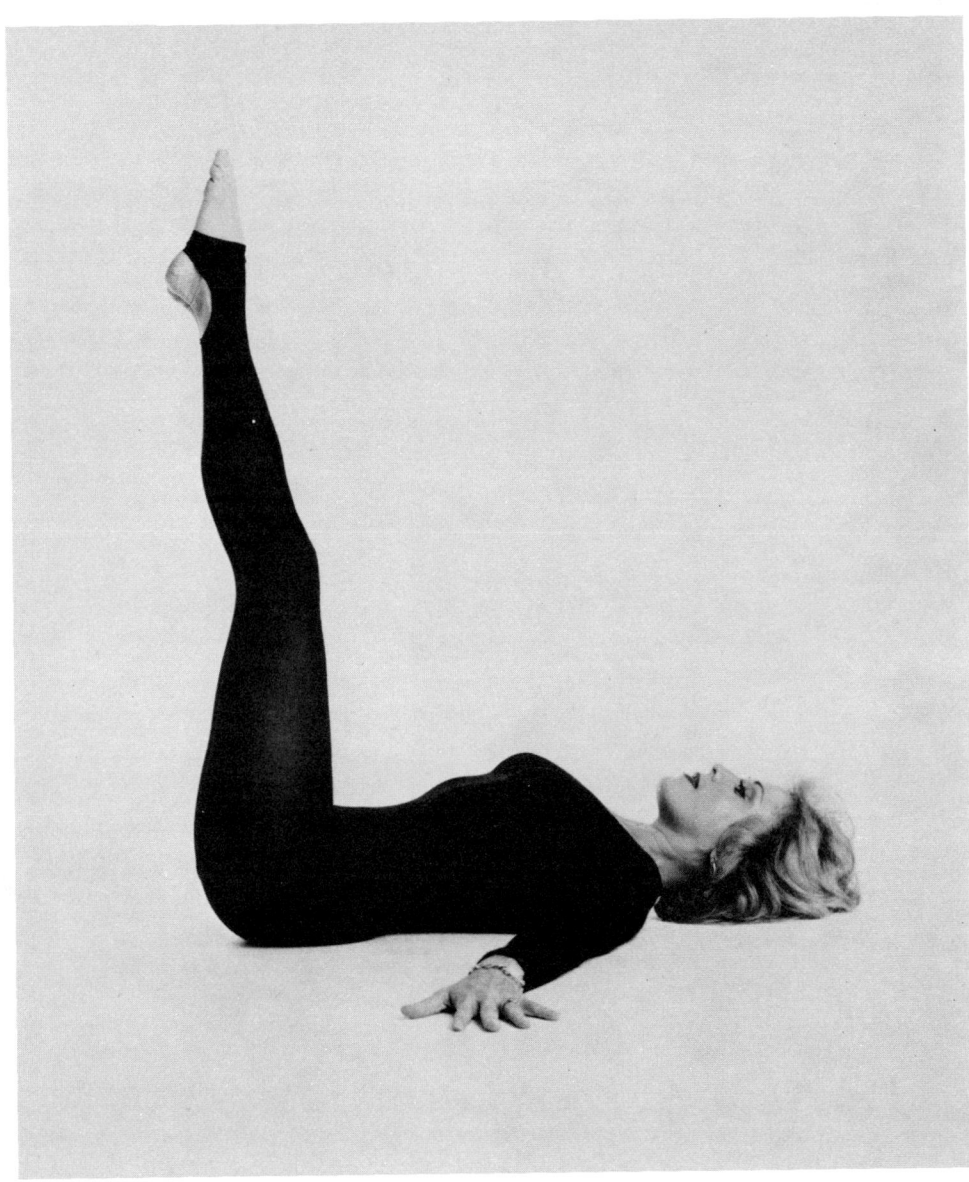

8. To further flatten and strengthen your stomach muscles, stay on your back and do leg raises. Try raising *both* legs—simultaneously and slowly—to a vertical position on a count of 5, then lower them on a count

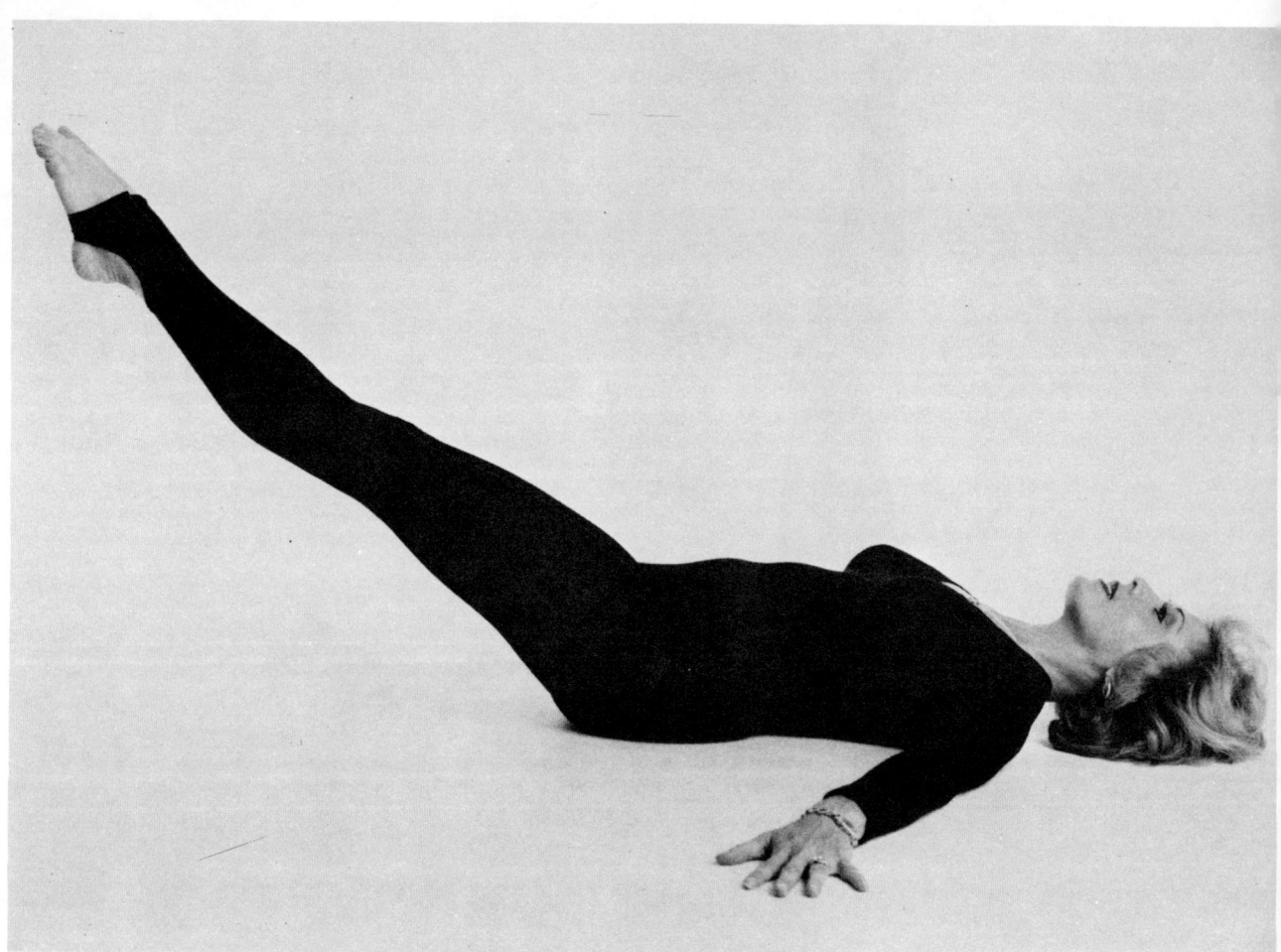

of 10. Ah, sweet torture! Start with 5 today and add one every day until up to 10 or 15 a day. If you *really* want to put your abdomen to the test, do these leg raises as described, but never allow your legs to touch the floor when you lower them. Stop 2 inches before you reach the floor. You'll tire much faster doing it this way, and I suggest you try it only after having worked up to 10 daily. If you have lower-back problems, do this one with your hands, palms down, tucked under your hips.

LET'S GET STARTED 25

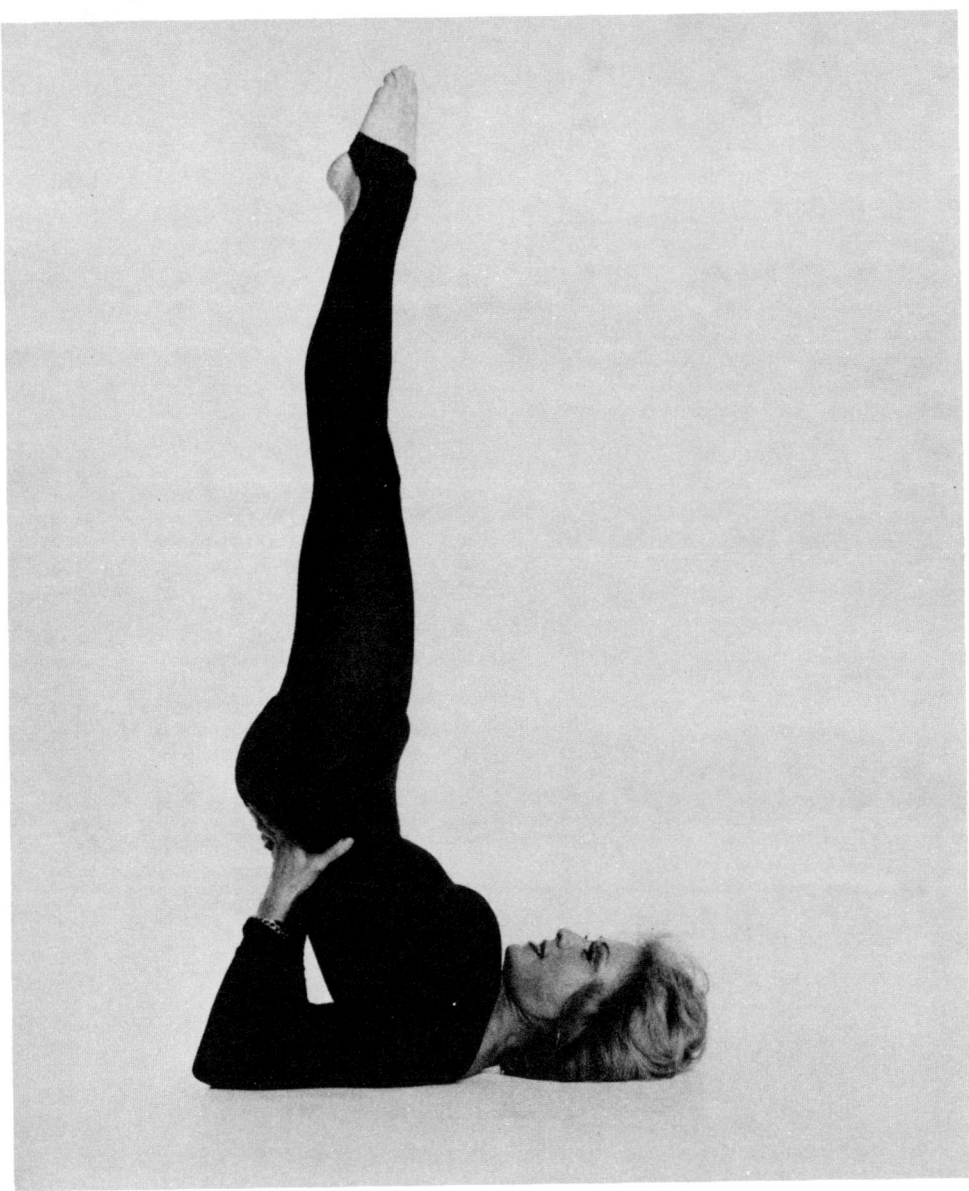

9. The shoulder stand. Raise your legs and hips toward the ceiling and hold yourself up by propping your hands at the back side of your hips (the same position you assume for the bicycling exercise). With legs held straight and toes pointed, try holding this position for 2 minutes. It brings the blood to the thyroid as well as the head, and leaves you with a rosy complexion.

The fourth day.

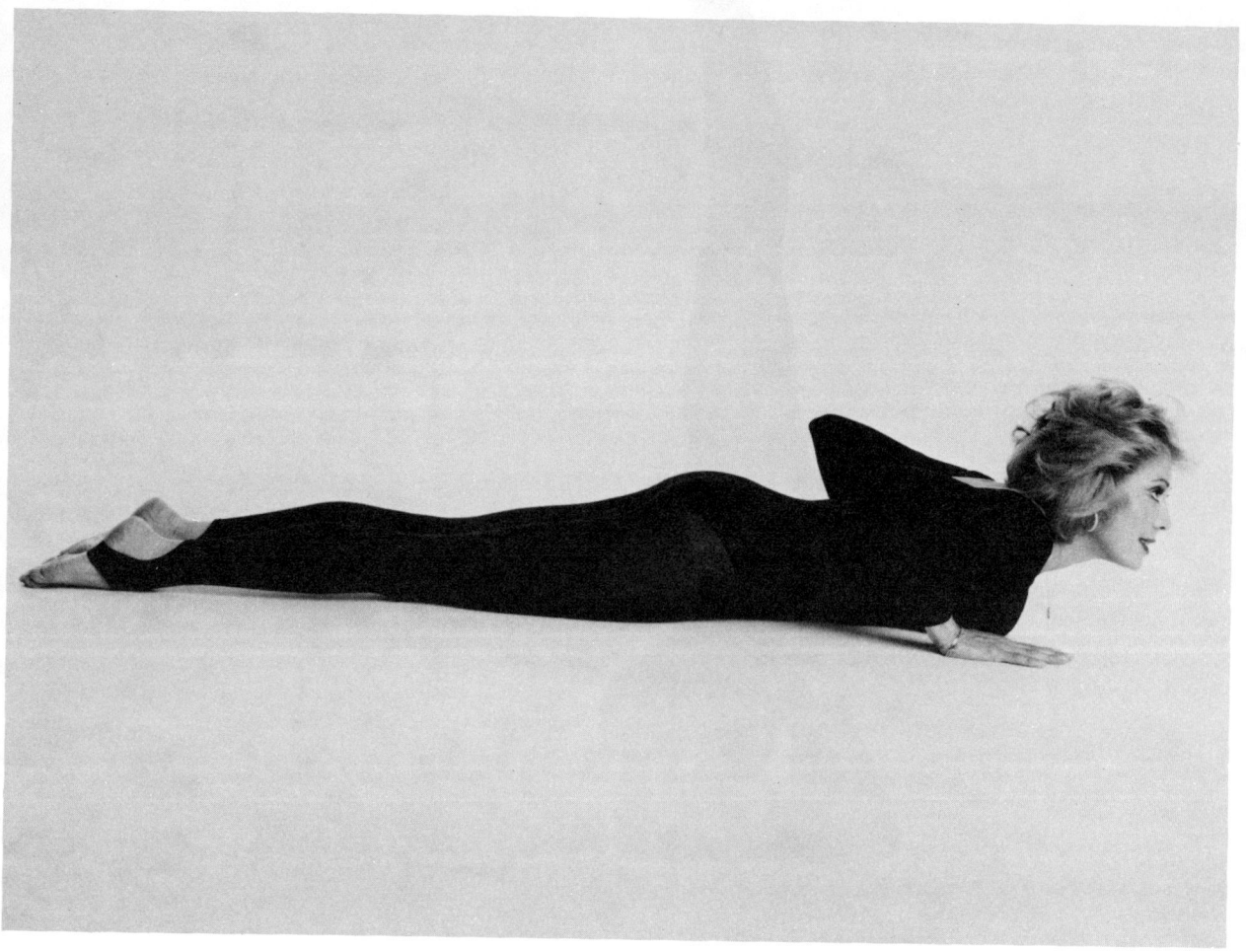

10. Today you're still on the floor after your shoulder stand. Now, do what is called "the cobra." Roll over on your stomach and place your hands, palms down, beside your shoulders, as though ready to do a push-up. Slowly raise your head and upper torso by pushing up with your arms.

LET'S GET STARTED 27

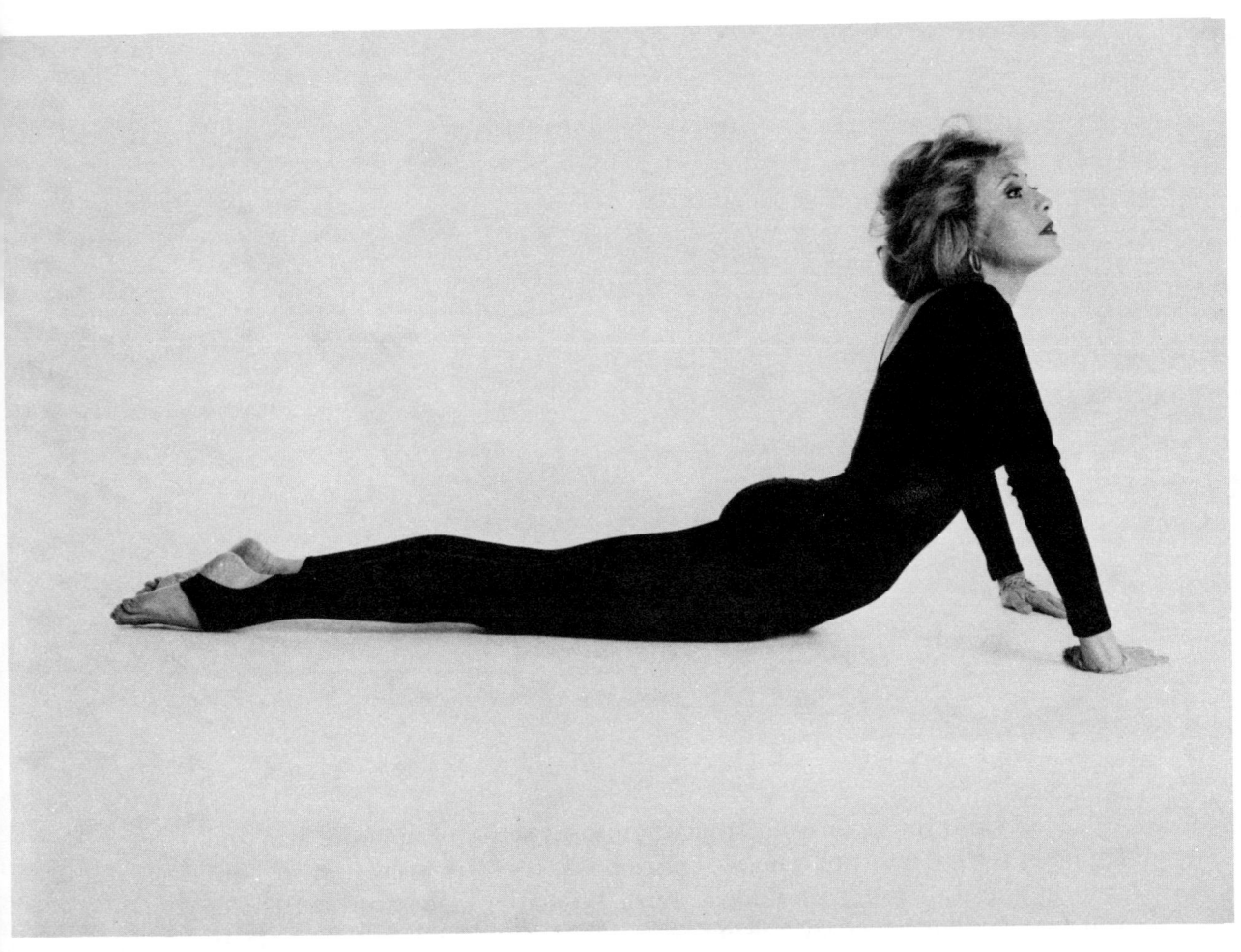

Arch your head back and try to get a good arch between your shoulder blades by turning your palms inward, which will make your arms pivot into a winged position. Now slowly lower yourself back to the floor while pivoting your arms back to the original position beside your body. Try to do this exercise slowly and slinkily, like a snake. Raise and lower 5 times today and add one more every other day until you're doing 10 a day.

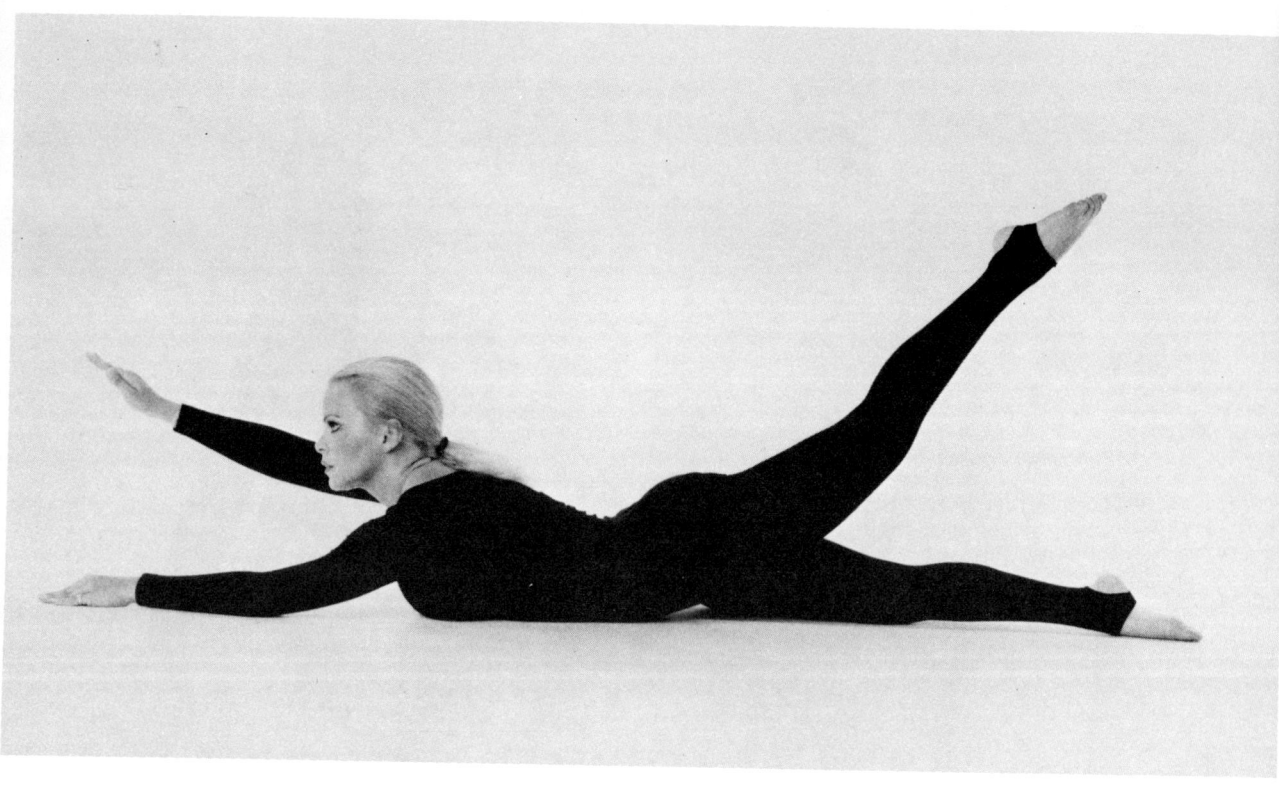

11. While you're on your stomach, a short series of opposite arm and leg raises is a good way to tone the entire body. Lie with arms stretched out straight ahead of you, palms down. First, raise your right arm in front of you, while simultaneously raising your left leg. (You won't be able to raise them very high.) Hold for a count of 2, then lower. Now reverse the procedure and raise the left arm with the right leg. Do each side a total of 3 times. Then raise *both* arms and legs at the same time. While your arms remain up and out in front of you, flutter your raised legs over and under each other several times. Then lower both arms and legs and rest a moment (you'll need it) before repeating the "double raise and flutter" action. You needn't increase the number of times for this exercise in following days. Three of the opposite arm and leg raises and 2 of the raise-and-flutter make a sufficient daily stretch.

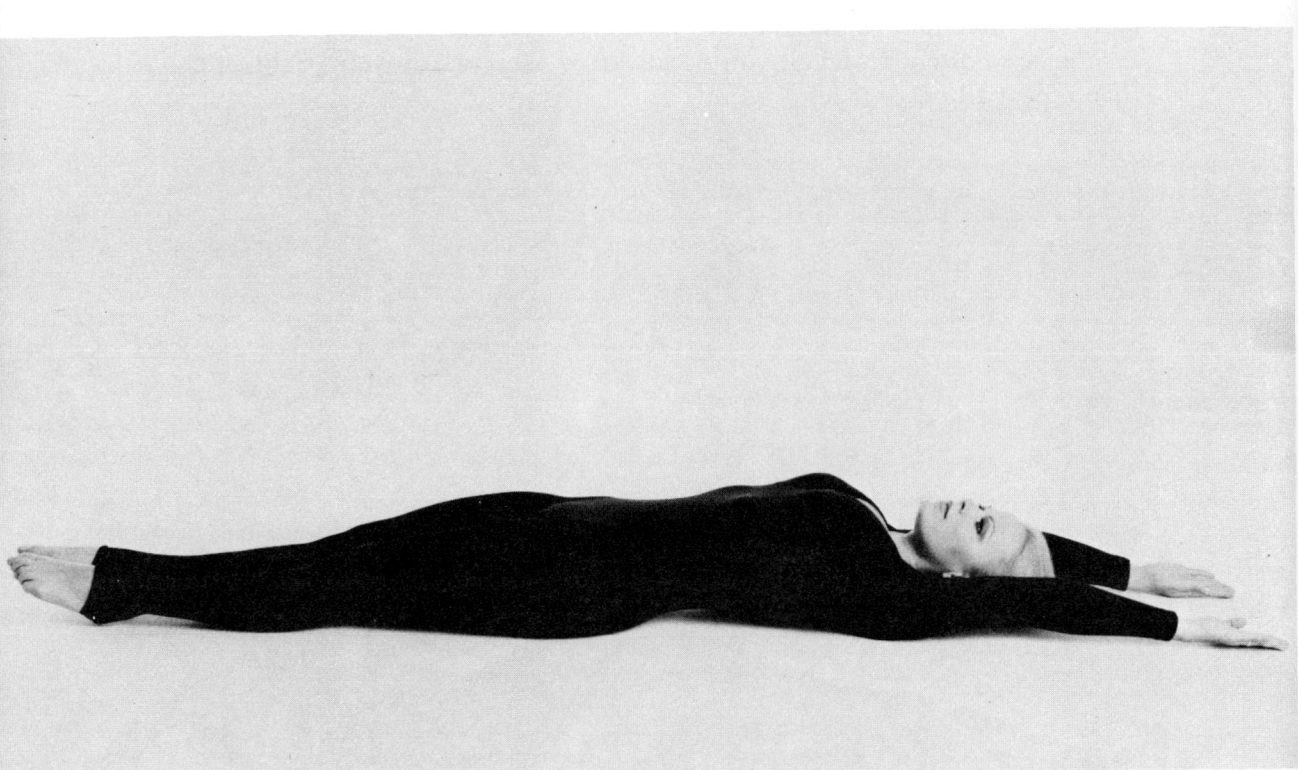

12. The last exercise for today is so simple it shouldn't be called an exercise. Just roll over on your back and lie flat, then try to tighten your stomach and touch the small of your back to the floor, while you deep breathe in the way I've already described, and relax for a minute.

The fifth day.

You have quite a nice little regimen of exercises now, and the last set you'll pick up today works specifically to reduce and tone the hips and legs. The three new exercises are to be done on both sides, but rather than turn over so often, I suggest you do all three exercises on your right side, then repeat all on your left.

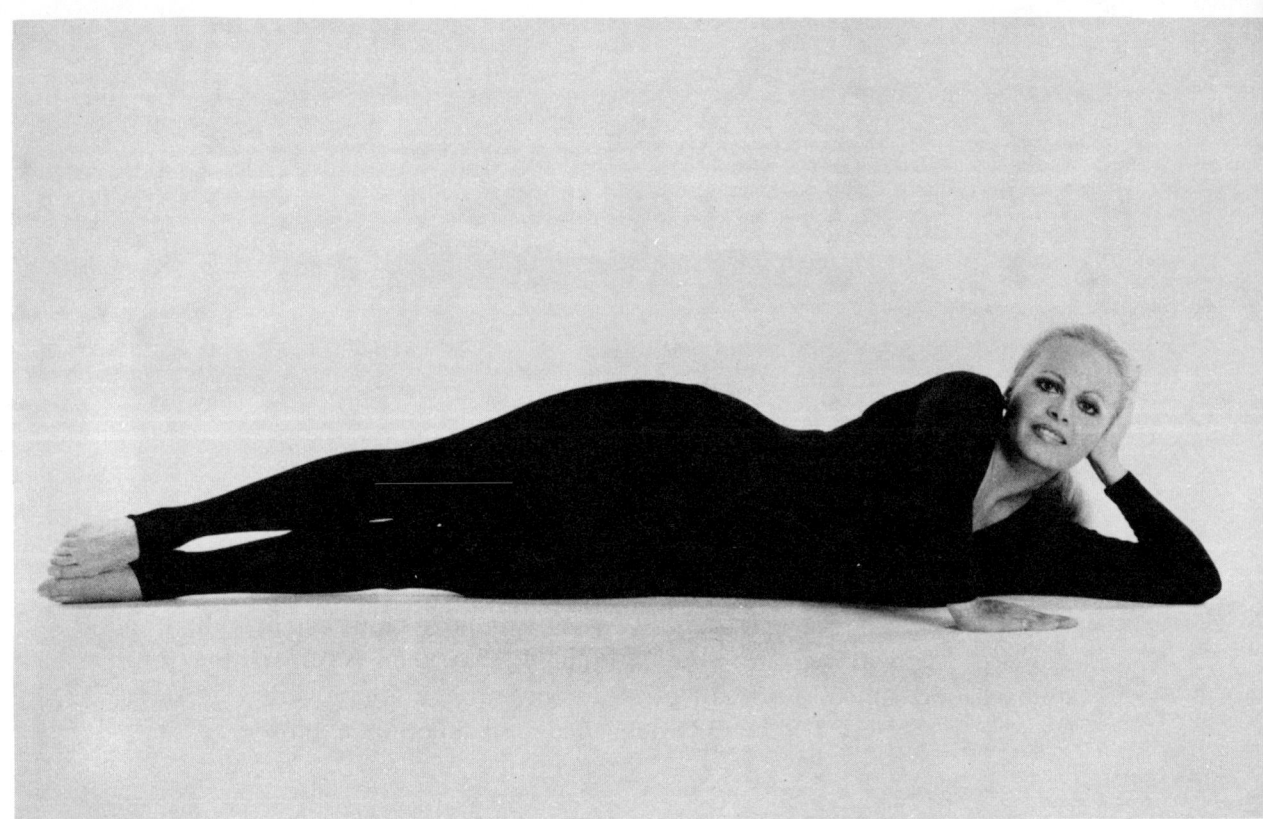

13. Vertical scissors. Lie on your right side and prop up your head with the right arm. Place your left hand on the floor in front of you for balance. Now, keeping your ankle toward the ceiling instead of your toes, raise your

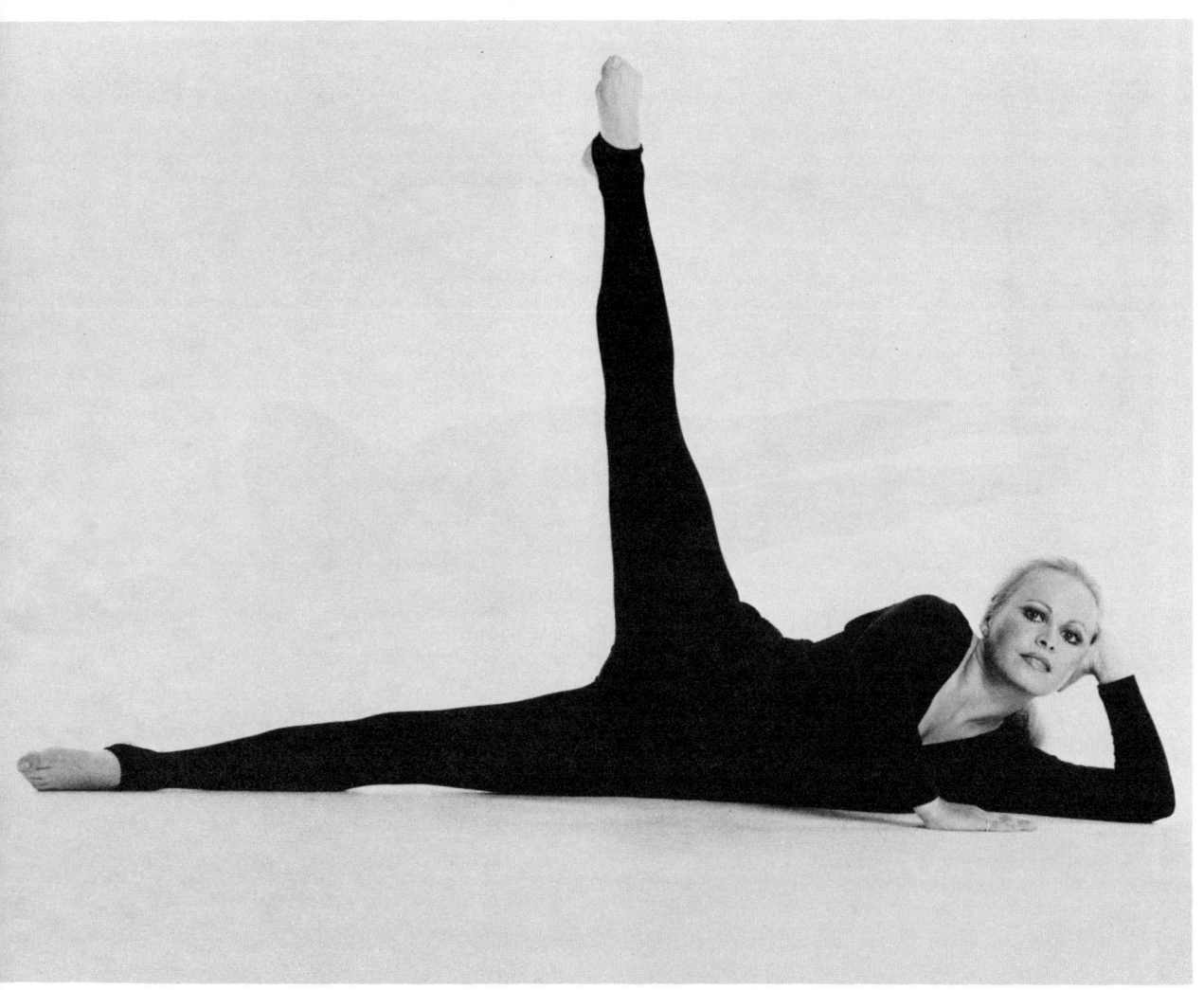

left leg as high as possible, then lower to touch your other leg. Raise and lower 20 times, then repeat on your left side. (The reason you "pigeon-toe" your foot: it results in more use of the muscles on the outside of thigh and hip.)

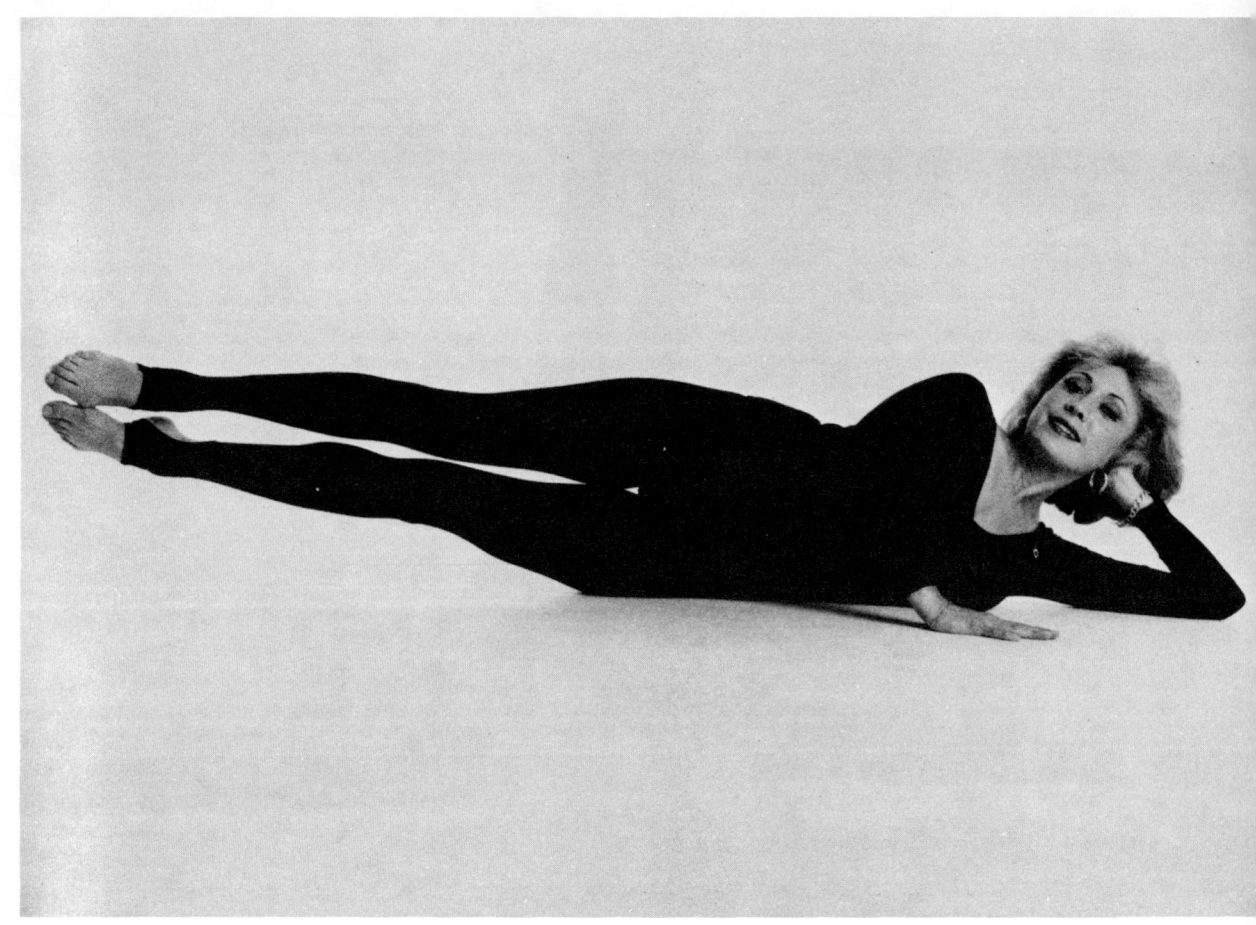

14. Horizontal scissors. Lie on your right side and balance with your left hand in front of you . . . same position as the vertical scissors. Raise

LET'S GET STARTED 33

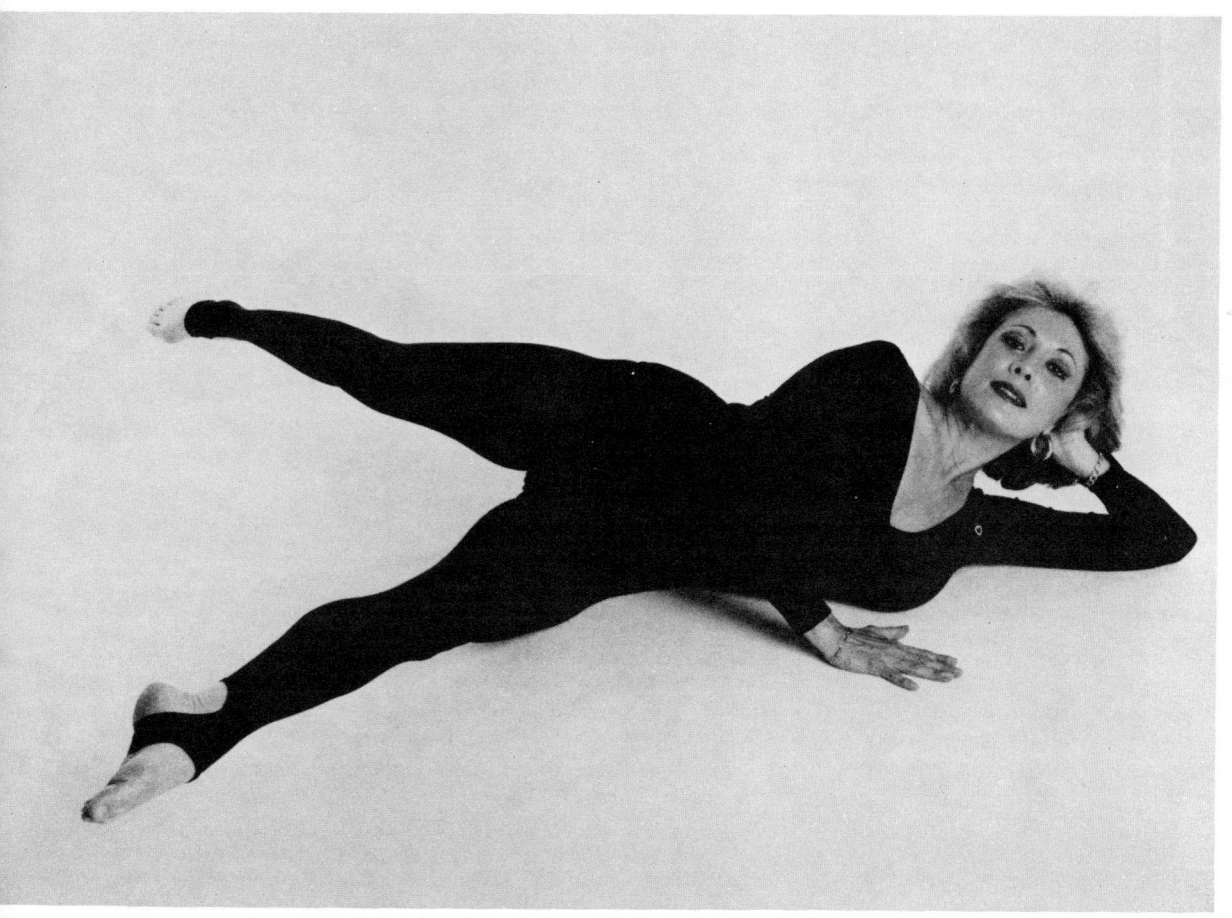

both legs 6 inches from the floor and move them back and forth in a scissors motion. Do this vigorously, 20 times, then repeat on left side.

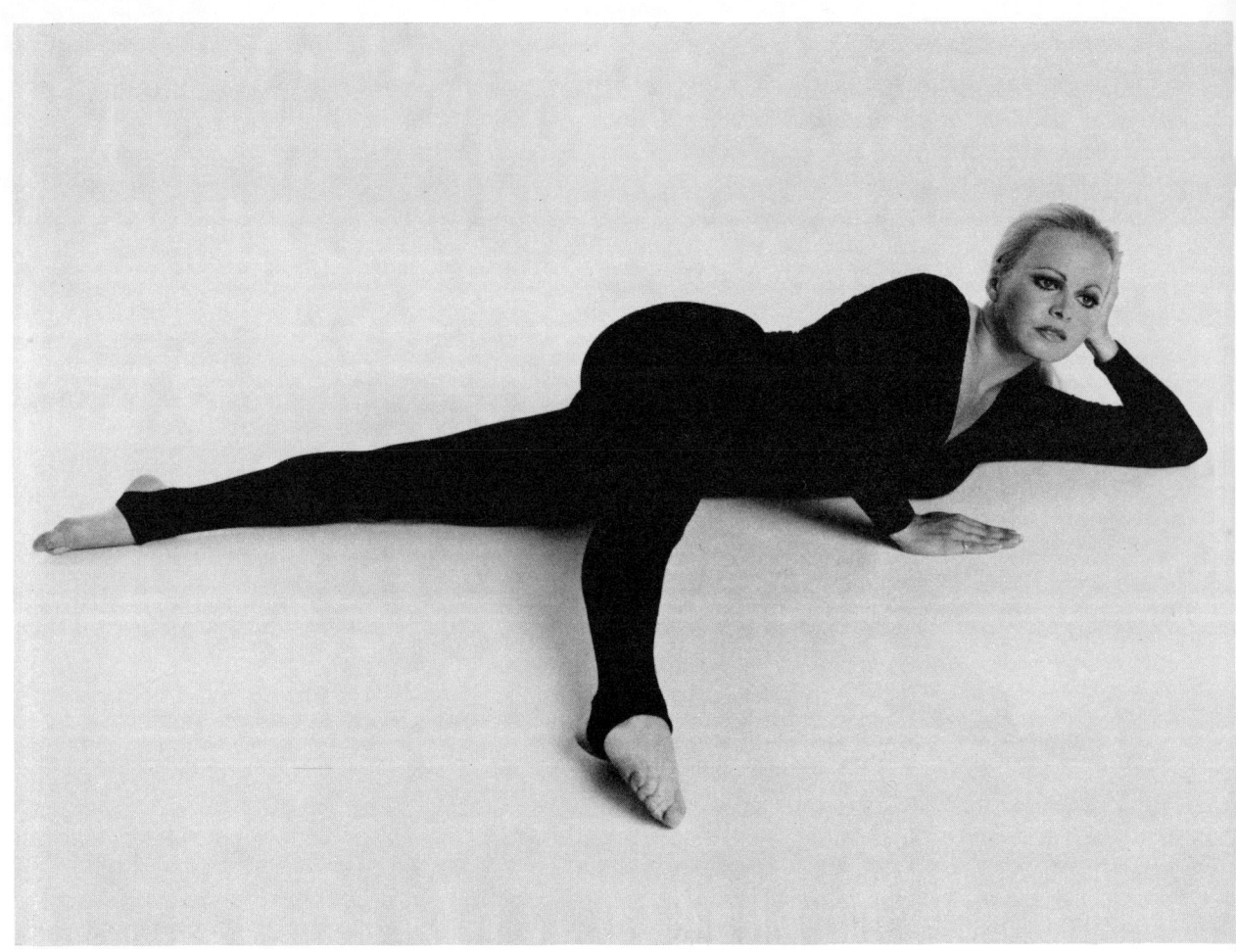

15. Leg swing. In the same position, on your right side, keep your right leg stationary and straight while your left leg does the work. Lift your left leg and bring it forward to touch the floor in front of you, then swing

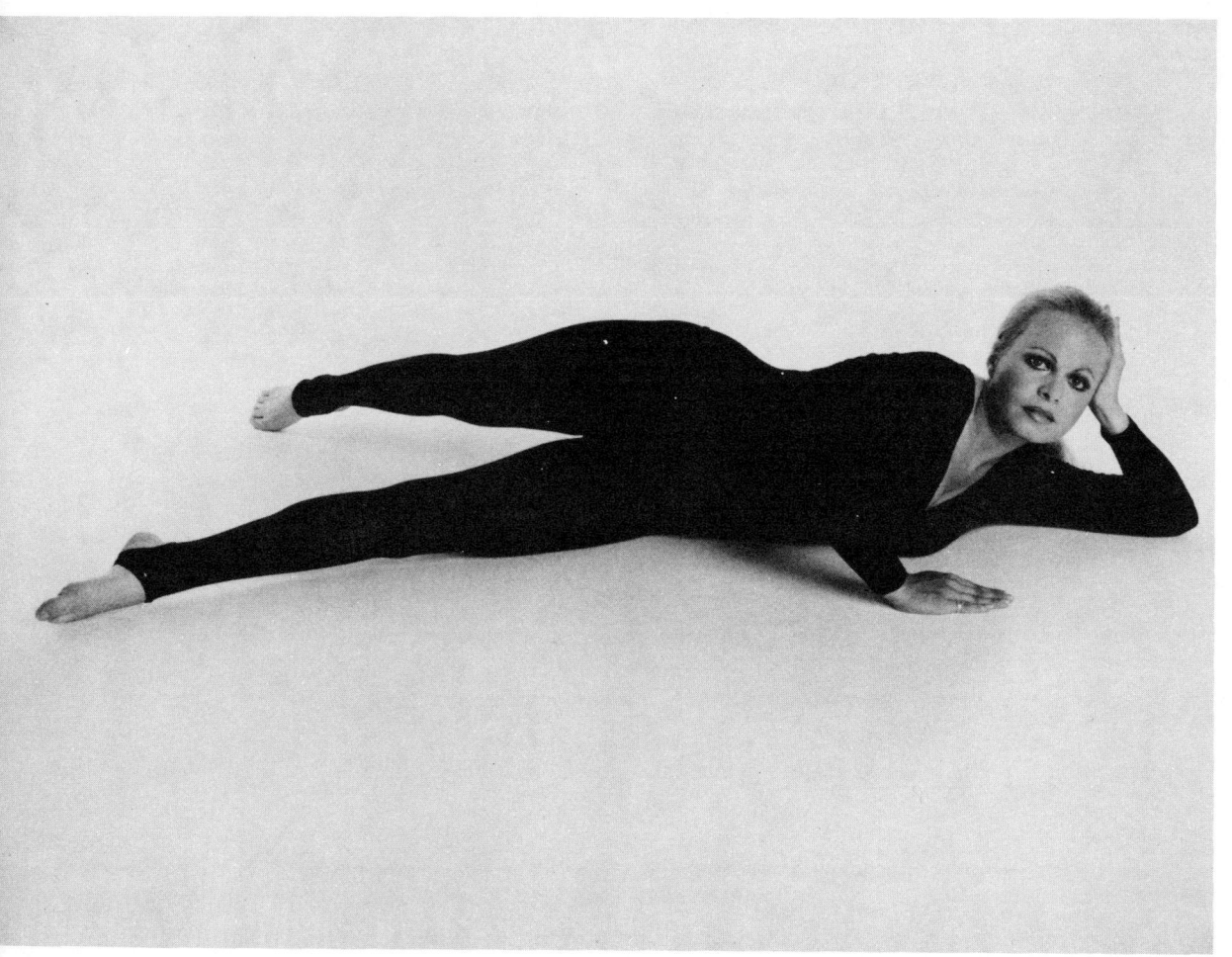

it up and backward in an arc to touch toes to the floor behind you. Swing the leg forward and back this way 20 times. Repeat on left side.

If you do these fifteen exercises every day, you'll be in tip-top shape.

3
Skin-the Big Wrap

Assuming you've lived for three days on only water and the juices of fruits and vegetables, you are now clean inside. The fast was a lot easier than you'd thought, you probably look better already, and you most certainly should feel better.

Now we have to get you gleaming on the outside.

Let's talk about skin for a minute. Skin is important. It's the largest organ of your body, weighing about seven pounds, and its nineteen square feet is distributed so that it wraps you up rather neatly. Without skin, you'd appear as a bunch of bones and muscles, in which case nobody could learn to love you. If *nobody* had skin, the whole human race might die out from total disinterest in each other.

Appearance is the least of it. The skin is like a blanket in that it helps maintain your normal body temperature, which is in the area of 98.6. And it acts as a sort of third kidney, ridding your body through the pores of all the gunk stored up inside you. It is a living, breathing organ, and as such, must have oxygen. Your outermost layer of skin is shed approximately every two weeks, and the condition of the new skin emerging from beneath depends on the sort of nourishment you've been giving your body.

How can you nourish skin? Simply by feeding it, both internally and externally, what it is made of. Skin is 98 per cent protein; the rest is made up of fats, necessary to keep skin from drying and wrinkling.

We also need carbohydrates to nourish the skin. When eaten with protein (and they need each other to work properly), carbohydrates make energy and the protein builds cells. I think many of us are confused about carbohydrates. There's a big difference between the refined (in white flour, pastry, etc.) and the natural carbohydrates found in whole-grain bread, fruits, and vegetables. So when you need energy, don't eat cake—eat an apple.

I seldom go to a market that I don't see a mother bribing her child to behave with the promised reward of a cookie. There go the kid's teeth, along with his skin and a few dozen other vital parts of his body. Why not, "Be quiet, darling, and I'll buy you some nice fruit."? Early conditioning sets the pattern for our reward systems, and I wish my mother had taught me that if I finished my dinner I could have an orange or an apple.

Joyce wants me to be certain I've straightened you out on carbohydrates. People think of them as "starch and sugar." True, but it's the *refined* flour and *refined* sugar we must delete from our diet. Did you know that sugar is addictive; the more you have, the more you want? Table sugar is nothing more than a refined carbohydrate (really a chemical) and has no nutritional value whatsoever. In *The Answer—Preventive Medicine,* authors Cleave, Campbell, and Painters write, "There is convincing proof that obesity, coronary disease and high blood fats are caused by overconsumption of sucrose and white flour." It's been estimated that 90 per cent of overweight patients are suffering from excessive fats in the blood caused by sugar and white flour.

Because the skin must work so hard to rid you of impurities, it's important to help it by flushing the system via the intestines. For this, you've got to eat roughage, or fiber . . . whole grains, nuts, seeds, fruits, and vegetables. I have a salad almost every day to take care of this, plus vegetables, of course, but to insure that I get my fiber, I buy fresh bran by the bag and keep it in a jar in the fridge. Every morning I sprinkle it on granola—or if I don't feel like granola, I take a huge tablespoon full of bran and squeeze some honey on top so that it'll go down. Otherwise, it sticks to my tongue. Joyce has taught me to take water immediately after and to drink plenty of water during the day. Without lots of liquid, bran would make a paste and stick to the intestines, reversing the desired reaction.

Incidentally, honey is an excellent substitute for refined sugar, but watch it if you're overweight—one tablespoon of honey contains 100 calories, even more than sugar.

So we need fiber and natural carbohydrates and protein, but the greatest of these is protein. An under-supply will flab your muscles and age your skin in nothing flat. (No pun intended.) A rule of thumb for the daily needed amount of protein is 1 gram for every 2 pounds of body weight. As as example, if you weigh 110 pounds you should have up to 55 grams of protein. How do you get this much? In the Appendix, there's a chart of various foods and their protein content, given in grams, which will make it easy for you to calculate.

But remember that fish, fowl, eggs, and dairy products are the best sources, and easier to digest than red meat. You're figuring on a big steak tonight, right? Wrong. Meat *is* a good source of protein, but it's loaded with fat, additives, and preservatives—all those poisons we're trying to get rid of. If you must have it occasionally, cut off all fat; a small steak can have 450 calories. And I suggest you never eat meat after four o'clock in the afternoon, because it's so difficult to digest that some of it doesn't digest at all. These horrible little leftovers putrefy in the intestines and their toxins enter your blood stream. Not good for a beautiful skin. I might also mention that the red meat I *used* to eat at late dinners gave me nightmares.

It can cause more than nightmares. Seventh Day Adventists, who abstain from eating meat, have been found to have (as published in the *Journal of American Medicine*) 40 per cent less coronary disease, 400 per cent less death rate from respiratory disease, 1,000 per cent lower death rate from lung cancer, and 50 per cent less dental cavities among their children. Put *that* on the spit and cook it!

Joyce says that a small amount of animal protein will give the skin color and a look of vitality, but begs you to skip red meat most of the time. If you are absolutely dying for it, here is Joyce's list of substitutes for the protein in one ounce of red meat:

>2 tbs. cottage cheese
>
>>or
>
>1-inch cube of solid cheese
>
>>or
>
>1 ounce of fish
>
>>or
>
>1 ounce of fowl
>
>>or
>
>2 shrimps
>
>>or
>
>1 cup of milk-base soup
>
>>or
>
>1 egg
>
>>or
>
>1 glass of milk

Food containing total proteins include all sprouts, mung beans, lentils, etc. You can grow your own sprouts from any type of grain.

A recent report from the McGovern Committee on guidelines for the United States asserted that Americans eat too much meat. Argentina is another country where meat consumption is high, and they and we have the highest incidence of cancer of the colon. If you've stopped smoking and *that* makes you feel better, try avoiding meat for two months and you won't believe the sense of well being—and the fantastic improvement of your skin.

I repeat, don't forget bulk—to chase digested (and *undigested*) food out of your system. Bush people in Africa eat lots of grain and seldom have problems with the colon. Remember that elimination of food should take place within twenty-four hours. I'm sure you wouldn't like to be confronted by a steak, chicken, or fish that had been sitting on your kitchen counter for three hot days. Well, that's what happens inside you if you don't keep food moving through. You could even develop diverticulosis (herniation of the intestinal lining), a painful condition that can lead to something as terrible as a colostomy (surgery of the colon, after which the patient eliminates into a container worn externally). Joyce keeps talking about balance; I think of it as "moderation in all things," a bit of advice penned by the Roman playwright Terence a couple hundred years before Christ.

Which leads me to the subject of overeating. You can be just as malnourished when you eat too much (and are of course overweight as a result) as when you eat too little. The answer is a combination of Joyce's battle cry of "Balance!" with my admonition of moderation. You really are what you eat, and an abnormal devotion to food, especially sugar and starches, can cause the skin to bloat and to become very sensitive to pressure. Test your own by pressing your cheek with a finger. If it turns red, knock off the doughnuts. You probably have excess waste material in your lymph glands—a fact that may not shake you up unless you understand that this will cause skin disorders.

So apply the information you've just learned with your own intelligence and get into the habit of eating properly. Vegetables (raw, if possible), salads, whole grains, nuts, seeds, and fruit. If you eat *properly,* you will never again have to go on a weight-reduction diet . . . a considerable bonus in addition to a beautiful skin.

Here are some handy hints about the combination of foods. Protein and starches eaten at the same meal can cause flatulence. Do not eat vegetables and fruit at the same meal because together they cause bloating. *Do* combine vegetables and protein. Fruit should always be eaten alone—a few hours before or after a meal—or as a complete meal, preferably in the morning. Fruit *may* be accompanied by nuts, which are not an animal protein but are considered as fruit of a tree. Melons should be eaten totally alone; melons are unique in that they do not combine well with any food, even other fruits.

If you would like a specific guide to a diet for your skin, here is the high energy diet Joyce has taught me. It gives optimum nutrition and energy, with the least calories. You should, of course, check it out with your family doctor, as I hope you have done with any diet you've ever tackled. You'll lose weight or at the very least stabilize your weight, and notice a surge in energy. And remember, if you want to look your best for the rest of your life, then stick to this intake for the rest of your life.

JOYCE VIRTUE'S DIET FOR SKIN NUTRITION

Morning: A cup of herb tea, sweetened with honey if you like. (Honey is high in pantothenic acid, an important B vitamin, but as you've been warned, high in calories.) Peppermint, camomile, or maté tea—all are great when you've just wakened. If you *must* have coffee, use a little raw milk to neutralize the acid. Or instead of tea, a glass of fresh fruit or vegetable juice, mixed half and half with water to cut acidity. For added nutrition, protein, and vitamin B, stir into the juice a teaspoon of brewers' yeast, debittered. It should always be taken in debittered form. (Joyce says brewers' yeast causes gas in some people, so start with a teaspoon at first and gradually build up to 2 tablespoons a day. Brewers' yeast is most easily digested in pineapple or tomato juice.)

Breakfast: If you didn't have juice on arising, have fresh fruit for breakfast. You can mix this with yoghurt (plain, not the fruit type, which contains sugar). Yoghurt encourages a healthy intestinal tract which, I keep telling you, shows up in your skin, fast.

or

The "or" is important because, remember, you shouldn't combine fruit with anything else. So instead of fruit, you might prefer one or two poached eggs, with toast made from whole-grain bread. And one very small pat of butter.

Regardless of what I eat for breakfast, even a cheese omelette, I always have Dr. Jacobus Rinse's formula for a healthy heart. (I have reason to worry about my heart because my father, a doctor, died at the age of fifty of a heart attack, and I know I may be prone to coronary disease.) By itself, Dr. Rinse's recipe will get you through until lunchtime. Joyce says Rinse's formula is imperative if you are on the Pill or have had a hysterectomy. In either case, your chances of heart disease or a stroke are elevated.

DR. JACOBUS RINSE'S FORMULA FOR A HEALTHY HEART

- 2 tbs. brewers' yeast (debittered)
- 2 tbs. lecithin
- 2 tbs. raw wheat germ
- 1 tbs. bone meal

Mix ingredients until thoroughly blended. To 2 tbs. of the above mixture, add 1 tbs. of soy oil or unrefined safflower oil and mix again. Eat this with yoghurt and/or honey, or applesauce, or on top of cereal. Joyce's husband, Nick, eats it with peanut butter—his sole contribution to this book.

Midmorning: Fresh fruit *or* a glass of freshly squeezed fruit or vegetable juice, mixed half and half with water.

Lunch: If you haven't yet had fruit, a bowl full of different fresh fruits, with yoghurt and raw nuts—unsalted cashews, almonds, or walnuts. Nuts that have been roasted have had their enzymes destroyed. Raw nuts are the one food that combines well with fruit.

or

A salad, made of raw vegetables, tuna, shrimp, or egg. Add alfalfa sprouts or mung bean sprouts. As a dressing use lemon juice and olive oil . . . the oil best for your skin. An alternative dressing is made with apple-cider vinegar, which is a good stomach clarifier, and soy or safflower oil. The oil provides the fat necessary for a healthy skin, but as a change, you might like the following non-fat salad dressing. Put in the blender ½ cup of pot cheese and enough non-fat milk to make a good dressing consistency. Add seasonings to taste—paprika, garlic powder, dill, for example.

or

If you are jammed with work and can't have lunch until late, make it the big meal of the day. Perhaps fish, vegetable, and salad. Then have a light dinner.

Afternoon: Fresh fruit and yoghurt. Or fruit and nuts. Or a glass of freshly squeezed vegetable juice. In the afternoon, do not repeat your midmorning snack. And check the calorie chart.

Dinner: Fish, cooked in any way except frying. Garnish it with yoghurt and lemon juice. Or chicken or turkey, both of which have one-third the calories of beef—and a lot more protein, ounce for ounce. Treat yourself to a baked potato a couple of times a week. Potatoes are not as fattening as commonly thought—the average size has only 80 calories. It's what you put *on* it that counts up calories. Try yoghurt instead of butter. Or cottage cheese instead of sour cream.

or

You can always switch lunch and dinner, having your heaviest meal at noon. Cottage cheese and vegetables are great for dinner, and you'll sleep better.

Bedtime: You'll also sleep better if you have a glass of milk before going to bed. Or kefir, a liquid yoghurt. (See Chapter 11 for the kefir "skin shake.") Calcium is a good nerve and muscle relaxant, and the older we get the more calcium we need. For B vitamins, add brewers' yeast to your milk —or any juice you enjoy. If you don't like the taste of brewers' yeast, substitute a B complex capsule.

People often ask Joyce for her "beauty secrets." She says she has none, that a beautiful skin isn't found in a jar of cosmetics; instead, it's available to anyone who follows the techniques she's learned in twenty-five years of research. If we nourish ourselves properly, our skin will reflect the achievement. Supple, youthful skin is the result of healthy physical and mental condition. As Joyce often says, if we spend twenty-four hours a day growing old, we owe ourselves thirty minutes a day to grow younger.

We've already given you the vitamins you should take every day. Specifically for your skin, Joyce says that you should add to these pills 20 mg. of zinc daily. Zinc is a natural nutrient, a metallic element you can buy in pill form at your drugstore. Joyce says you can ingest zinc in food form by eating brewers' yeast, bone meal, all beans, wheat germ, fertile eggs (get these at a dairy or HFS) and the seeds of pumpkins and sunflowers. Zinc means growth; without it, we would be dwarfs. Lacking zinc, hormones won't properly metabolize, you'll have an imbalance of proteins, your calcium and magnesium won't be assimilated correctly, and in addition to all of that, Joyce tells me, you'll have a problem with assimilation of vitamin B_6. With this sort of hassle, resulting from a zinc deficiency, it stands to reason your skin will suffer. It's likely to deteriorate into dry, scaly patches, much like psoriasis. In his research on aging, Dr. Benjamin Frank has stated that a deficiency of zinc interferes with the formation of the nucleus, as well as both RNA and DNA.

Guess who's going to explain RNA and DNA to you? Me. Having had a doctor as a father and now married to one, I've always been interested in medicine, and I paid attention in school. I can remember learning in biology class about RNA and DNA—and thinking at the time what wonderful words the letters stood for. Something you could throw around at a dinner party and impress people. Just because I know how to pronounce them doesn't mean you have to, but when I tell you they are, respectively, ribonucleic acid and deoxyribonucleic acid, you'll understand why they're commonly known by the letters.

Let me go back to my biology class. When we're conceived we are only one cell, and this cell is constructed of the acids RNA and DNA. Within these acids are all the components that will dictate our final height, the color of our eyes, consistency of hair, how long we'll live, even the likelihood of a coronary attack. It's a wondrous thing to see under a microscope—all sorts of ladders and sundry tiny forms. This first cell divides and divides over and over again, until a human being is complete. There will be several references to RNA and DNA in the book, so I figured it should be explained right now.

DOWN WITH DRUGS

I've told you what you should eat and drink to effect a beautiful skin. I'm now going to tell you what you should avoid, and almost all of it can be summed up in one word—DRUGS. Joyce's prescriptions for your health and beauty do not contain as much as a gram of any drug. As a doctor in Naturopathy, which can be defined as "health without drugs," she is adamant in her advice that all drugs be avoided if possible. If you follow the recommendations in this book, you'll seldom be ill. If you are, drugs might well be prescribed by your doctor, but then you'll be taking them only as a last resort. When*ever* you're sick and/or take drugs, you and your skin age more rapidly—a fact your friendly druggist doesn't noise around the neighborhood.

Another enemy of the skin is the common aspirin, which millions of people take indiscriminately. Aspirin does not cure anything—it simply relieves pain. And sometimes by relieving pain, it stops the symptoms by which a doctor can diagnose an illness. Know that aspirin is a strong medicine. So strong that it will show up throughout your system—even in your hair—within a matter of minutes. When drug companies advertise that their aspirin gets into the system *fast,* they're not fooling. It has no nutritional value, and when it hits an empty stomach, it can cause holes in the lining. (How'd you like your doctor to tell you, "Put two holes in your stomach and go to bed."?) That's why aspirin should never be taken on an empty stomach, and why aspirin tablets should be mashed before swallowing, most particularly for children.

In addition to stomach lesions, aspirin can cause ringing in the ears, allergies, and skin rashes. If that isn't enough to discourage you from popping aspirin every time you have a twinge somewhere, let me give you further facts—facts printed in scientific journals. Brace yourself. Aspirin has been found to cause gastrointestinal bleeding, and anemia. It has caused anaphylactic shock (advanced hypersensitivity), asthma, and hives. It can damage the kidneys, is potentially toxic to a baby within the womb, and can affect a woman's ability to deliver her baby.

I'm going to drone on about aspirin just a bit more and give you a case history about how it can affect the skin. Back in 1965, two women were admitted to a Connecticut hospital, both suffering from bad cases of psoriasis—which is something red and blotchy and scaly that you never want to happen to your skin. Both women, coincidentally, had complained of hearing problems, and since psoriasis does not affect the hearing, doctors ran a check. It was discovered they had been using the same ointment to relieve the itching of psoriasis—an ointment with a high content of the same acid prevalent in aspirin. Aware that high doses of aspirin were suspect as a cause of hearing loss, the doctors checked this salicylic-acid level in both women and found it to be extremely high. Their conclusion: the acid so prevalent in aspirin had actually penetrated the skin.

The Pill is included in this group of recommended taboos. I'm no doctor, but I'm sure you've read of the multiple side affects of the Pill, many of them disastrous—strokes, cancer, even death. I read about a girl married to a pre-med student who advised her to take the Pill. So did her doctor. She developed breast cancer, had a mastectomy, and died at the age of twenty-four. Less serious was the girl I saw in Schwab's drugstore, her face a mass of large and ugly brown spots. She told me it was caused by the Pill. Among other things, the Pill can cause deficiencies of the ovarian, adrenal thyroid, and pituitary glands.

For years, the Pill was shipped to druggists in large boxes containing hundreds of packets. There was one warning slip of the possible side effects per box, a slip customers never saw. A new law makes it mandatory that drug companies include a warning slip with each packet. But how many women bother to read it? Or if they do, how many heed the warning? It's the same thing with the cautionary note on every package of cigarettes. People tend to ignore it.

Certainly, the Pill's advantage in controlling population growth is a fine thing. But there are a lot of negative aspects, and I'd suggest you give these serious thought. If your doctor won't show you his own copy, get the Physician's Desk Reference at the library and read all the possible side affects of the Pill—and aspirin, too, while you're at it. Then decide for yourself if that's the type of birth control for you. After all, other options are available.

PLAY IT SAFE WITH YOUR SKIN

Watch for new spots on your skin, brown or black, bluish-black, red, or scaly. They'll probably go away, but *if they don't,* and particularly if they grow larger, do see a dermatologist. He'll look you over and probably say, "These thirty-two are freckles and those two are moles, and I think I'll take this one off." Relatively few people die of skin cancer, probably because skin cancer is easily detected in its earliest stages, and can be removed painlessly.

CARE OF THE SKIN

Let's assume you've been persuaded to do all of nature's things that are good for you—and scared away from the unnatural, negative things. We'll now teach you how to take care of your skin from the outside.

It's been said that everybody has at least one feature that is good and should be enhanced. Without proper modesty, I must say that my own is my skin. It was blessed by (1) the Norwegian complexion of my mother, (2) the Scottish complexion of my father, and (3) the incident of having grown up in Oregon, where there's a strong tendency to rain. My skin is very fair and very thin—you can see the faint outline of blue veins all over my body. Its good texture does not make me adorable—let's just say it's a nice skin.

SKIN—THE BIG WRAP

For now. Somehow, the young believe they'll never get wrinkles. The fact is that *at age sixteen the skin begins to deteriorate with loss of moisture.* From then on, unless you take care of it, it's downhill all the way.

So I do try to give it tender loving care, and have particularly since I've known Joyce. Mine is what might be called a normal skin—except for a penchant to perspire from my face much too freely, a habit that gives me trouble with makeup, but I'll get into that later.

The very first rule of skin care is to keep it clean. Did you know there's a term for "city skin"? Dermatitis urbis is used by dermatologists to describe the epidermal condition of city dwellers. It's hard to believe how much soot, grime, and for all I know, smog, gets into exposed skin. I believed it when Bill and I went to Montreal on our honeymoon. I'm not knocking Montreal. It's a lovely city, but it's a *city*. After a couple of days there my eyelids began itching like crazy. Bill thought I had a foreign object in my eye and told me to use eye drops. "Or maybe it's your mascara," he said. Well, there was nothing *in* my eyes, and I was using the same mascara I've always used. So when we came home I asked Joyce about it and she said, "Now you know what dermatitis urbis is." As she has pointed out to me, if polluted air can destroy the marble sculptures of ancient Greece, if it can seep into the prehistoric caves of France and damage the painting on granite, just think what it can do to your skin. Skin is a tough organ, protecting us against heat, cold, and dirt, but it can't fight the battle all by itself. Urbis can cause such unlovely things as dry skin, premature wrinkles, pimples, infection, dandruff, and blackheads.

But even if you live on a farm, your skin must be kept clean because it's constantly expelling impurities from within your system.

SKIN CLEANSERS

It isn't necessary to cleanse your face in the morning if you have given it proper care the preceding evening. Every night, remove your makeup and clean your face with a natural vegetable oil, one that does not contain mineral oil. Then follow with a skin freshener to remove the oil. A good natural freshener is the mixture of 1 ounce of apple cider vinegar to 8 ounces of water—especially good for teen-agers. Use with a cotton ball, and keep refrigerated.

A more thorough cleansing of the skin is recommended once or twice weekly. Place your face over a steamer or a sink full of hot water, holding a towel over your head to capture the moisture. An easier method is the application of a warm towel to the face.

When the skin is warmed, the pores open and are ready to be stimulated with a good facial scrub. Here's the one Joyce uses every morning, leaving it on while she showers. Mix equal amounts of oatmeal, honey, and almond meal, apply to your face and scrub gently, with particular attention to the problem areas of chin, nose, and forehead. Rinse off, then close the pores with a splash of cold water.

A good scrub for oily skin is a simple paste made of cornmeal and water.

An excellent facial mask for closing the pores before application of makeup is made of avocado and cucumber. Mash an avocado, dice a cucumber and put into the blender until smooth. This mask should also be rinsed off with cold water. After patting your face dry with a clean towel, apply a good moisturizing cream, preferably one containing vitamin E.

Dry Skin Cleanser

You can make your own with equal proportions of glycerine, plus lanolin *or* vegetable oil—and petrolatum. Except for the vegetable oil, all can be purchased at a drugstore. About petrolatum, or petroleum. I want to tell you that when Joyce advised me to put it on my face, I screamed. "Petroleum goes into a car!" I said. "Why would I put that stuff on my face?" She explained that petroleum is refined one way for motors, another for external application to human beings—as in good old Vaseline, which is labeled "petroleum jelly." Oil, said Joyce, is important to our lives in more ways than one. And it comes from the earth, doesn't it? I had the same horrified reaction about zinc, which is used to coat iron and steel. But zinc is also from mother earth and necessary for our well being.

If your skin is dry, make sure your astringent does not contain alcohol —which will dry your skin faster than the sirocco wind. Skin fresheners do not usually contain alcohol, but to be on the safe side, read the labels of any freshener or astringent you buy.

Oily Skin Cleansers

These are all made with detergents, so washing with a mild soap will have the same effect as an expensive cleanser touted for oily skin.

SKIN—THE BIG WRAP

THE SKIN SHAKE

This is excellent for any type of skin, and you should drink one every day as a meal in itself—not with other food, or you'll gain weight.

- 6 oz. of kefir plain
- 1 to 2 tbs. of brewers' yeast, debittered (remember the advice re brewers' yeast. Start with 1 tsp. for 2 weeks, then gradually increase to 1 or 2 tbs.)
- 1 fertile raw egg (dairy or HFS)

or

Fruit. Strawberries, pineapple, or banana. *Half* a banana if you tend toward tubbiness. (Fruit *or* egg, not both)

Whip it all up in your blender.

We've given you two concoctions—Rinse's formula and the skin shake—recommending both daily. Joyce has brought up the important point that both contain brewers' yeast, and warns that you will ingest too much brewers' yeast if you take the skin shake and Rinse's formula on the same day. So, you can have one *or the other* every day. Your choice depends on whether you prefer treatment for your skin (drink the shake) or your heart (take Rinse's formula).

Whatever care we give our skin, we must remember that it is aging. Don't take umbrage at the inference you are an old crone. The entire human body begins to age at birth, and as I've already pointed out, skin begins losing moisture—therefore deteriorating—after sixteen years. Studies have indicated that vitamin C—or lack of it—has a great deal to do with aging. We need vitamin C from the moment of conception. Vitamin C is necessary for formation of collagen, the substance that literally holds us together. You've already read that you should take two tablets of 500 mg. each day (you can make it three if you like, adding one more at bedtime), but I'm stressing this point here because I'm about to broach the subject of aging skin.

FACIALS

At what age will facials help keep skin from aging? Sixteen to forever. Facials are important, and well worth the time they require. If you can't afford having them done by a professional, I have a batch for you to try—then you can choose your favorites.

Just don't *wait,* as did one aging film star, whose name I can't mention because she's still floating around. I saw this woman a few years ago at an Academy Award ceremony, and mentioned to a friend how lovely she looked. Said friend had known her for years, and told me *why* the actress looked so well. It seems she parts her hair about an inch back from the hairline around the face, and brushes that section forward. Then, mind you, she selects small bunches of hair in back of the part, braids each one, and pulls them back very tightly from her face. Then she combs the front hair back over all this tugging and lifting mechanism that is making her facial skin seem so taut. So there she was, beautiful as of yore, smiling away with a migraine headache.

A SKIN TIGHTENER

This one will do the same thing for you without giving you a migraine. It's great for preventing wrinkles and is a good nutrient for the skin. Any wrinkles you already have will be minimized, and if you use this tightener frequently, you'll stave off further disaster.

Mix the beaten white of an egg with a little sweet cream so that it is spreadable. Apply to thoroughly clean skin and leave on for 20 minutes. Remove with lukewarm water.

REJUVENATING MASK

This is for any type skin, which will have the feeling of silk after the mask is removed.

½ cup of rolled oats that have been soaked overnight in buttermilk.
Strain mixture through cheesecloth.

Apply to clean face and leave on 15 minutes. Remove with lukewarm water.

FACIAL MASK WITH FULLER'S EARTH

Mix ½ cup of fuller's earth (from DS or HFS) with ¼ cup of cornstarch and enough oil to make a paste. When I mention oil, unless otherwise specified, I'm referring to soy, safflower, or olive oil. Applied to the skin, this mix produces a tightening action, and takes dirt with it when removed with warm water. I specify warm water, because this mask gets rather hard and needs warm water to soften it for removal.

A substitute for fuller's earth is China clay (kaolin), available at pharmacies. Use the same formula, the same procedure.

DRY SKIN FACIAL

4 tbs. brewers' yeast
2 tbs. dry milk solids
Camomile tea, enough to make a paste

Apply to clean skin, leave on 15 minutes, then flush with cool water.

DRY SKIN FACIAL

Mix 1/4 cup of soy protein powder (at HFS) mixed with enough oil to make a paste. Apply to skin where it is dry or blotched, leave on 15 minutes, and rinse with cool water.

DRY TO NORMAL SKIN FACIAL

This is a mask rich in protein and natural oils.

1 avocado, thoroughly mashed
1 egg yolk
2 tbs. olive oil

Beat together in blender, apply to clean face, leave on 15 minutes, and flush with cool water.

FORMULA FOR DRY SKIN

(from Swedish Institute in Phoenix, Arizona)

1/2 cup sesame oil
1/4 cup avocado oil (HFS)
1/4 cup sunflower oil
2 fresh egg yolks
1 tsp. apple-cider vinegar
Few drops of perfume

Beat the eggs, mix oils in cup, and slowly add to eggs. Continue beating, add vinegar and perfume, and beat a bit more. (Keep it in a tightly covered jar in the fridge.) Apply for 15–20 minutes, remove with cool water.

The old line about egg on your face is, in actuality, a darned good idea. You've noticed how many facial treatments contain eggs. The reason is not only that the 4 grams of fat in each egg mix well with your own natural oils, but the lecithin in eggs helps to emulsify any mixture of oil and water. Further, lecithin attracts moisture from the air and then holds it to the skin . . . and you know how beautiful the English complexions are, inundated with rain and fog. Lecithin also improves skin because it improves the respiration. And when skin breathes easily, this tends to slow down its aging process.

FOR DRY AND SCALY SKIN

If your skin is extremely dry or undernourished, try a castor oil pack. First, open the pores with warm towels. Then make a paste of castor oil, powdered brewers' yeast, and add a touch of lemon juice (not more than $\frac{1}{2}$ teaspoon). Remove from the skin after 10–15 minutes and rinse with cool water.

The foregoing masks for dry skin are not an end in themselves. You must remember to moisturize your face before each application of makeup, and again at bedtime.

The following two facials for oily skin are to be applied before bedtime.

OILY SKIN FACIAL

Mix $\frac{1}{4}$ cup of corn meal and enough golden seal tea to make a paste. Rub gently over the skin and leave on for 10 minutes. Flush with cool water, then powder your face with cornstarch and leave on overnight. Powder only the oily areas—chin, nose, and forehead.

OILY SKIN FACIAL

The same ingredients used in the Dry Skin Facial on page 51—with brewers' yeast and milk solids—but instead of camomile tea, use 1 tbs. of lemon juice. After the cool water rinse, powder your face with cornstarch and leave on overnight. Again, powder only on the problem areas of chin, nose, and forehead.

Powdering with cornstarch, even without the facial, is beneficial to an oily skin, but only on nose, chin, and forehead.

THE SUN AND YOUR SKIN

I'm sure you don't have to be told that prolonged exposure to rays of the sun will fry, roast, bake, boil, and sizzle your skin. The damage is unrectifiable and therefore permanent. There are enough suntan lotions on the market to fill up eight shelves in any drugstore—some of them good, some not so good. The only way to choose is to look for one that contains PABA, or para-aminobenzoic acid. PABA is the best sun block available, and you should never be in sunshine for any length of time without covering the exposed parts of your body with PABA. Read the lotion's label before you buy. If you know you're susceptible to sunburn, Joyce suggests that before exposure you can also take PABA orally.

If you didn't know about PABA and have already gone and done it, looking and feeling like a cinder, I can give you many remedies.

I only wish I'd known about even one of these after I made my second visit to the Hawaiian Islands. The hotel doorman was a lovely big native with copper skin that absolutely glowed. Little Caucasian me, with the blue-and-white skin, said to him, "The first time I came here, I didn't get any suntan at all. How do you do it?"

He didn't say he tanned well because he had inherited a brown skin. He drew himself up with pride and said, "We Hawaiians don't use lotions. We go into the sea, come back to the beach to dry off for a while, then go back into the water. In and out, in and out, that's the way to do it."

So I did it that way, for hours. They had to pack me in ice and wrap sheets around me. They knocked me out with drugs to kill the pain, and took the arms out of two first-class seats on the plane so I could lie down. They took me off the plane in a wheel chair, and I couldn't move for a week. I was not only badly burned over 90 per cent of my body, the strain on my kidneys was extraordinary.

Don't listen to people who have a lot of melanin in their skin and tan naturally. (Not that they *are* free from sun damage. Dark-skinned people, including blacks, haven't as much warning as whites because they can't *see* that their skin is burning. There is more incidence of skin cancer in Hawaii than anywhere else.)

So you have a sunburn. Do *not* apply anything with oil in it to your skin. The recommendation for butter on a burn—any kind of burn—was a dangerous old wives' tale. With the heat emanating from the burn, oil will further fry your skin.

Do take a cold tub. It won't be easy. Because your skin is so hot, even mildly cool water will feel like ice. Lower yourself into it slowly, even if your teeth are chattering, and stay a few minutes until your skin has been lowered in temperature. After gently drying off, apply either buttermilk or 1 oz. of cider vinegar diluted with 8 oz. of water over all burned areas. Cider vinegar takes out the sting, and is particularly good if you've been in water containing chlorine, but be careful not to apply the vinegar too near your eyes.

Or, make a strong solution of tea from Cantor's tannic acid or theobromine, and apply on burned areas. Both have healing factors. (From now on, I won't remind you to look up unfamiliar items in "What's THAT?" Everything you need to know is explained in that chapter.)

Or, apply juice squeezed from raw potatoes.

Or, use the aloe vera plant. The juice of this wondrous plant, when applied to a burn, will stop the pain almost instantly, and help to prevent peeling. I once saw this applied to the scalded hand of an artist friend in Florida. She broke off a small branch from a plant growing in her back yard, and when she removed the torn leaf after a few hours, her skin was almost healed.

Another remedy to avoid subsequent peeling: mix equal amounts of buttermilk and mashed fresh tomatoes. This will help restore the skin's natural balance.

If your face is badly burned, give yourself a daily facial made with a mixture of buttermilk and plain old Quaker oats. Soak overnight ½ cup of oatmeal in 1 cup of buttermilk, then strain, apply to your face and leave on 15 minutes.

Or, mix sour cream with a raw egg—or yoghurt with a raw egg—and leave on your face for 20 minutes. The egg's protein repairs the damage of the ultraviolet rays.

Here is a recipe for any bad sunburn, particularly if you have blotched instead of burned evenly.

- 2 tbs. honey
- 2 tbs. lemon juice
- 2 egg whites
- 2 tbs. almond extract (not the type for cooking, but the pure almond extract not processed by chemicals—available at HFS)
- ½ cup of oatmeal that has been soaked for 1 hour (save the water from this)

Mix honey, lemon juice, almond oil, and egg whites, and add enough oatmeal to make a paste. Apply this to burned areas and allow it to remain for 30 minutes. Rinse well with cold water, then rinse with the liquid in which the oatmeal was soaked.

If you have been severely burned all over your body, it's a good idea to keep dunking yourself in cool baths. These are better than a shower, which is too much of a shock and pelting water on a burned skin can be painful. You can add 1 cup of aveeno to your tub, an oatmeal you can buy at drug store or supermarket. Aveeno is very soothing and helps remove heat from the skin. Do not envision lowering yourself into a batch of porridge—I assure you it will all go down the drain when you pull the plug. (Mix it well with the bath water—oatmeal can make a tub slippery.)

Now that I've told you how to avoid a burn and what to do about it if you get one, I'd like to suggest that you consider whether or not a suntan is worth it. The damage done by overexposure to sunlight when you are sixteen or sixty doesn't go away, and there's nothing you can do about it. When on the beach you seldom can see the extent of the burn, and it's only when you get home and take off your suit that you realize you've roasted yourself half to death.

So suppose your neighbor does play tennis every day and has a tan you envy. Or a friend looks sexy in white because she spends her leisure time stretched out in the sun (probably smeared with PABA-less oil, for heaven's sake). They will both look like prunes long before they *should* look like prunes. Is it really necessary to you to have the status symbol of a tanned skin? Who needs it? Think about the fact there's something very pretty and feminine about a pale skin.

It's your decision.

EXERCISES FOR THE FACE

Most facial exercises make you look utterly ridiculous, even a bit insane, and you might feel better about doing them if you keep away from mirrors while in the process. Following are nine suggested exercises for the face, which you should do five minutes every day. Try them when you're sitting at your desk or washing dishes. Any time when no one is looking at you.

A cautionary note: rapid movements are recommended. I work out in a gym four days a week, after work, and I've learned that any exercise done slowly builds muscles and therefore can give a negative effect. In contrast, if you exercise quickly you merely tone muscles. This relates to facial as well as body exercise, and is especially applicable in Exercise No. 1—holding a frown too long will result in permanent frown lines.

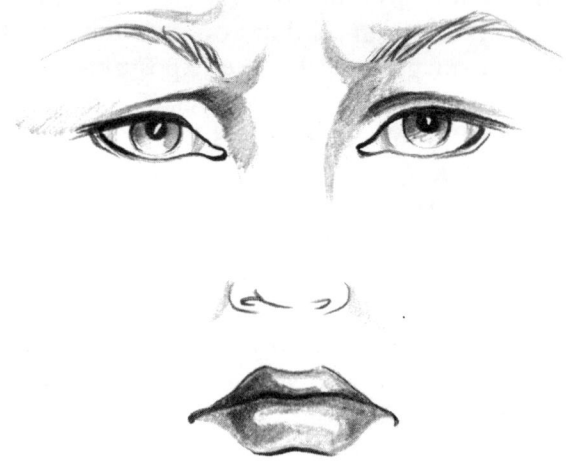

Exercise No. 1

Frown, then quickly open your eyes as wide as possible. Alternating these two movements will tone muscles surrounding the eyes.

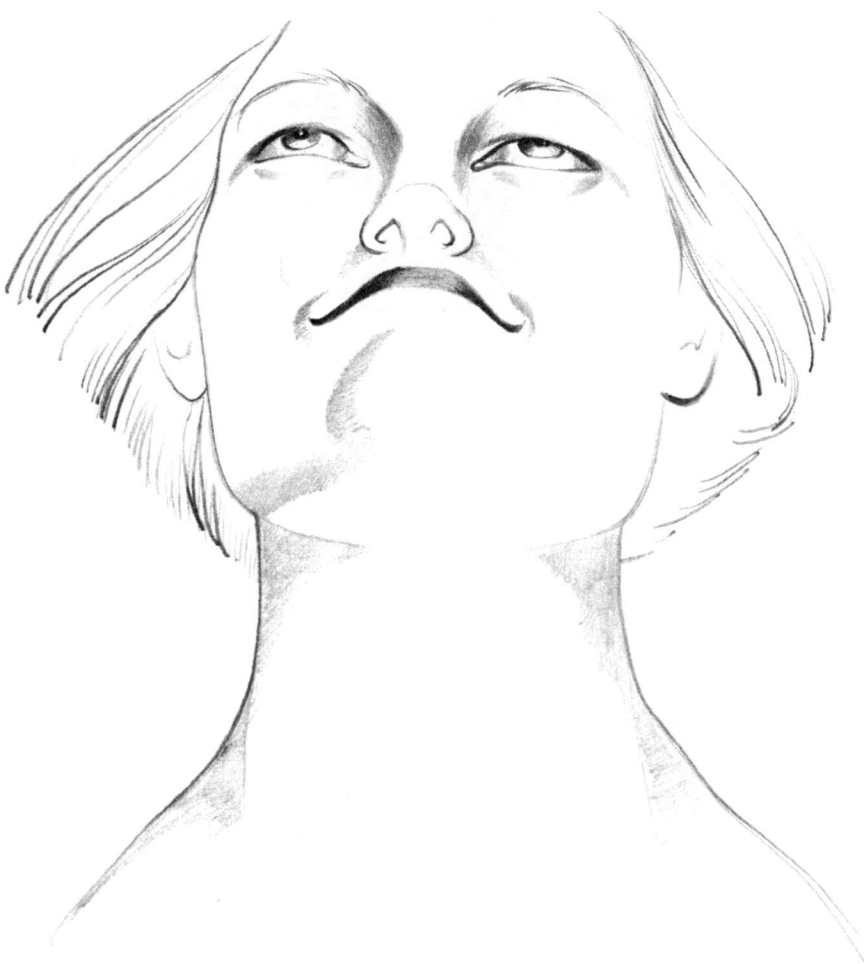

Exercise No. 2

To avoid a double chin and crepe neck, sit in a chair and relax. Tilt your head backward, way back. Strain to pull your lower lip over the upper one. Relax, then do it again. Got it? You can *feel* those muscles in the lower jaw.

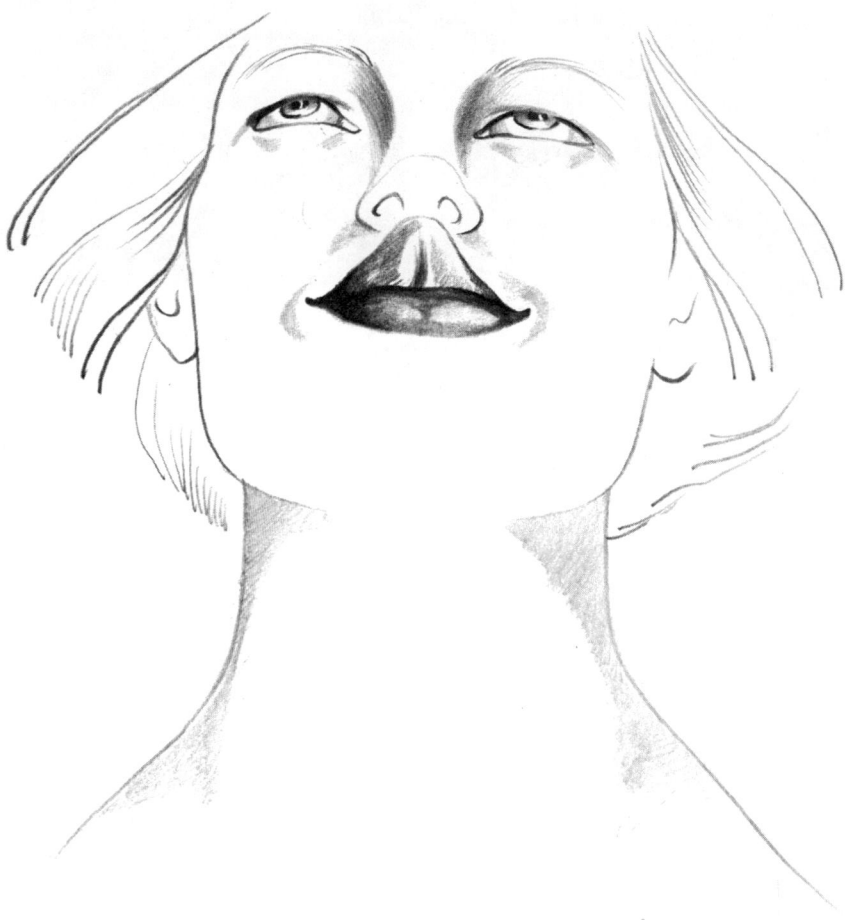

Exercise No. 3

Also for double chin, or the avoidance of same (I do this and the one above often, because both sides of my family tend to grow double chins), try to touch your nose with your tongue. Release, stretch again, release.

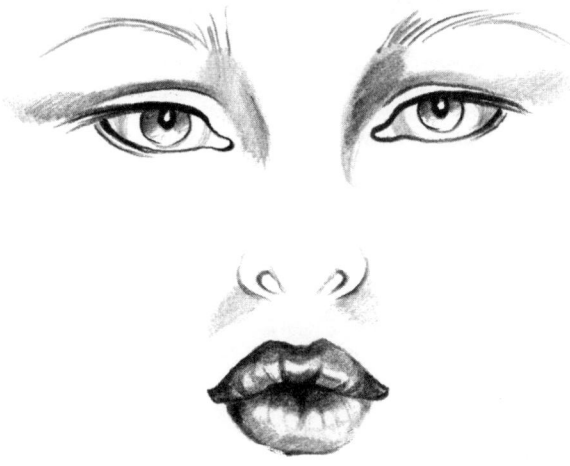

Exercise No. 4

For muscles adjacent to your mouth: form a kiss, a grin, a kiss, a grin—but exaggerate. Pucker up as though you were trying to kiss a prison inmate through the bars of his cage. Then grin so that your mouth is stretched as wide to each side as possible. Do this 10 times.

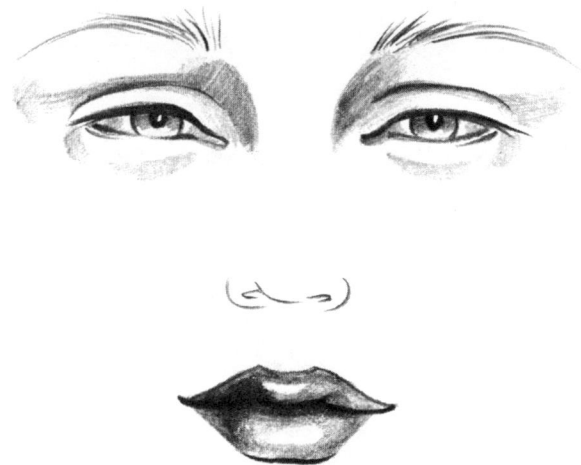

Exercise No. 5

Great for muscles around the eyes. Without furrowing your forehead or lifting your eyebrows, squint as hard as you can. Try especially to move the lower lids upward.

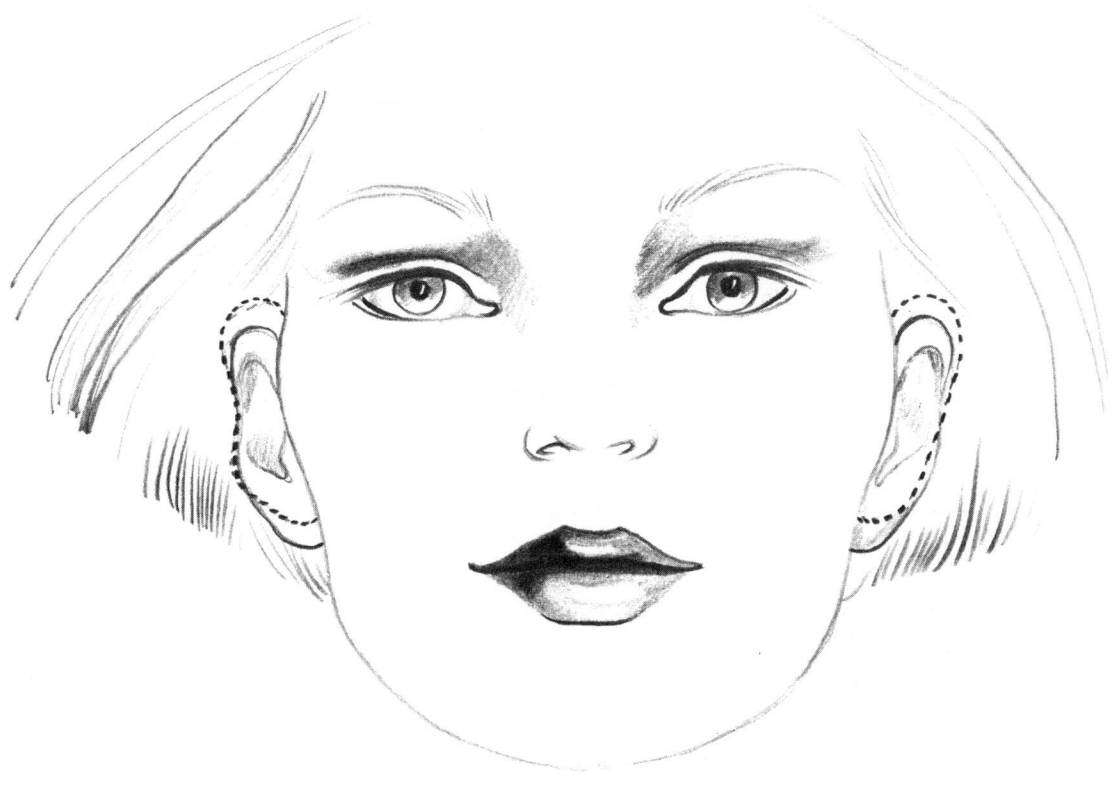

Exercise No. 6

Wiggle your ears the way your uncle used to do when you were a kid. You may not actually wiggle them, but the attempt will do wonders for your cheek muscles. Check this one in a mirror. You'll see your jaw and cheeks working like crazy, but probably not your ears. No matter. Your *ears* will never sag.

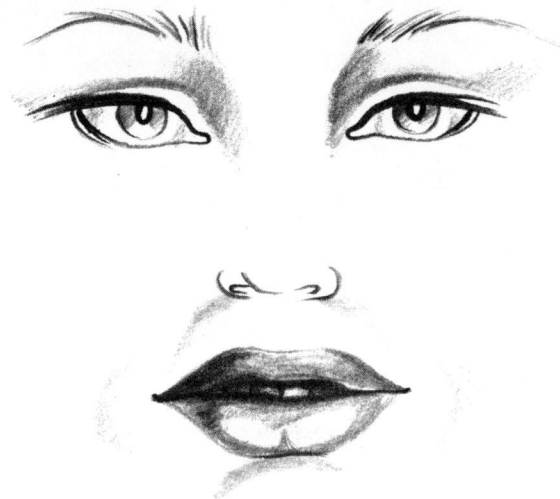

Exercise No. 7

Do a shoulder stand, as Joyce did on page 25, or a head stand. If you can't do either, lie on a slant board, head down. At the very least, lie on a bed with your feet up and your head tilted backward over the side. With blood going to your head, you immediately have circulation in your face and hair follicles. The after affect is a rosy blush.

Exercise No. 8

Flap your lips, by exhaling softly through them. You'll look like a whinnying horse, but the reward is a firm mouth.

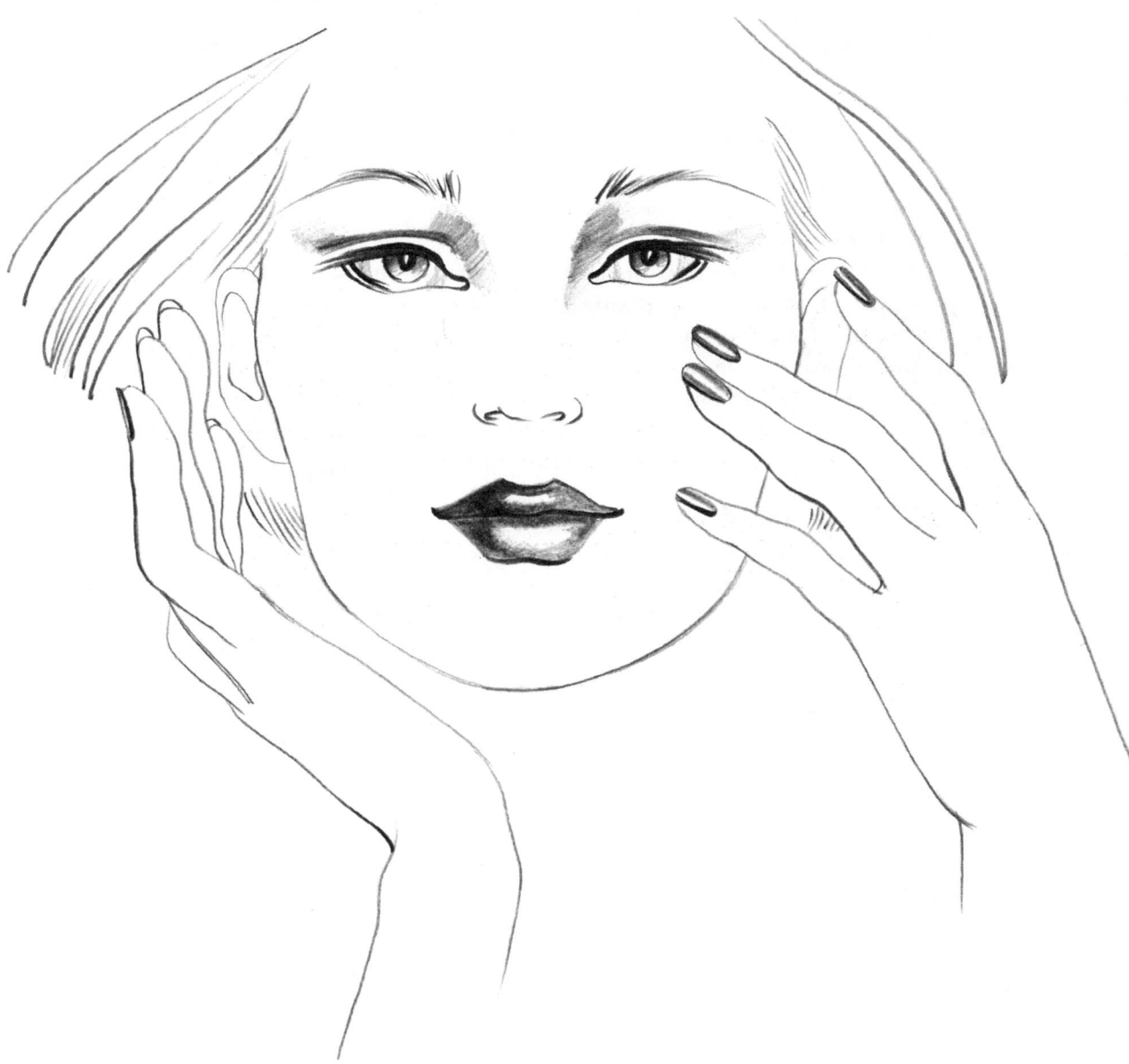

Exercise No. 9

Gently slap your face with your fingertips. Begin at the neck, move up to the chin, then cheeks. Careful not to do it too hard or you might break capillaries. This is wonderful for circulation; after a minute or so of slapping, you'll feel the tingle of the blood. It's a process included in every professional facial, and one you can certainly do yourself.

In general, you can make any silly face you want to. It's not true that making faces makes wrinkles. Just don't hold any pose for too long.

ACNE . . . THE BUM WRAP

What is acne?

1. It's embarrassing.
2. It's hard to get rid of.
3. It is, medically, an inflammation of the hair follicle within a pore. The pore fills with sebum, an oily substance that gives a pinkish-white color to the pore. If infected, it has a black center, forming a pimple. The acne lesions appear most frequently on the face, chest, and back.

Acne is not the same thing as a whitehead or blackhead. A blackhead is simply a dirty pore, usually enlarged, that can be cleaned out with steaming and a good scrub. A whitehead is a nodule in the skin, harder to remove than a blackhead because its source is often much deeper. If a whitehead goes very deep, all the way to the glands, it can form a cyst. You should take care of these immediately, so, as much as you might like to avoid the magnifying side of your mirror, keep a constant check. Whatever you do, do *not* pick. Particularly around your nose or upper lip. These areas should be cared for by a dermatologist—as should psoriasis, a severe scaling of skin accompanied by redness and itching. If you try to squeeze a blackhead or whitehead and don't get beneath it—particularly the whitehead—you can squeeze the infection further down into your skin. Squeezing at the areas around nose and upper lip has been known to send an infection to the brain.

It is important to keep hair away from any blemish on your face or neck. Hair can be dirty an hour after a shampoo, as you'll learn in Chapter 4, "The Mane Thing."

What causes acne?

1. Accumulation of toxins in the body, caused by allergies. If you suspect you are allergic to any food, avoid it for two weeks and observe how your skin reacts. The Japanese eat foods, such as seaweed, containing a great deal of iodine, but some people don't assimilate iodine well. That's why shellfish is banned from the diet of many acne victims.
2. It can be hormonal, which is why teen-agers are so often afflicted. At that age hormones are whirling around as though they were in a cement mixer, and when a teen-age girl frets and worries about her acne, the emotion only compounds the situation.
3. Stress, which in a way is akin to emotional upset.

What do you do about acne?

1. Use a good cleanser, morning and night.
2. Keep your hair healthy with frequent shampoos and good hair rinses.

SKIN—THE BIG WRAP

3. Drink a skin shake every day.

4. Clear your blood with a tea made of burdock root—1 oz. of burdock to 8 oz. of water, brewed 5–7 minutes. This is not a guaranteed cure, but most certainly helps to purify the blood.

5. Get your sleep. A good night's rest is beneficial because that's when the body heals and repairs itself.

6. Be sure to take your calcium before going to bed. Calcium calms the nerves and is effective treatment for any sort of trauma—including the trauma of an acne victim.

ACNE MASH #1

Golden seal tea: 1 oz. of golden seal to 8 oz. of water
2 tbs. brewers' yeast
Juice of ½ lemon

Make a paste of these ingredients and apply to affected areas. Let it remain for 15 minutes, then rinse with tepid water.

ACNE MASH #2

½ cup of fuller's earth
2 tbs. witch hazel

Mix and apply to skin, leave on for 20 minutes, then rinse with tepid water.

Both acne mashes reduce bacteria and remove excess oil.

And both should be kept away from your eyes.

To correct acne, you must increase your resistance to infection. Joyce suggests you add to your diet raw products of liver, pancreas, spleen, and thymus—all available in pill form, you'll be happy to know. You can get these by writing to Nutrydyn, 2210 Wilshire Boulevard, Suite 159, Santa Monica, California 90403. Or from a nutritionist—or an orthomolecular doctor, who is an M.D. treating only nutritionally. These people can best advise you about your acne problem.

If you've tried everything and the acne persists, we suggest you consult your family physician about high dosages of vitamins A, B, and C. Also, zinc should be considered.

I should mention here that a bad acne condition often persists after a woman discontinues the Pill. The Pill has not only caused metabolic disturbances, but has depleted the body of B vitamins. On the Pill you don't ovulate, and this causes a deficiency of progesterone. Along with the nutritional deficiency caused by the Pill, this can play havoc with the skin. If this is true in your case, you should have a complete metabolic evaluation and a therapeutic program including tissue supplementation with the particular glandular substances involved.

A note of hope. Acne is not terminal, so you're not going to fade out. But you *are* embarrassed, and for that I have a hint. I've noticed so many women who seem to habitually hold their hands over their faces to hide a blemish. This only draws attention to it. Deal with your embarrassment. The best way to handle the situation is to say to your friend/lover/whoever, "Would you look! I have this awful thing on my face and I feel terrible about it." You can bet they'll reassure you it's not all that bad. And then the subject is over and done with. It's just no use (and not sanitary) trying to cover up a blemish. In any way. I remember a girl in high school who covered every bloom on her face with the mark of an eyebrow pencil. I can only guess she hoped people would think she had outsized freckles. But it didn't work—she simply looked as though she had a batch of acne underneath a batch of brown marks.

Admit to the acne, do your best to cure it with the remedies Joyce and I have given you, and some day it's going to clear up.

PLASTIC SURGERY—IS IT FOR YOU?

It used to be that the incidence of plastic surgery was kept under wraps . . . like divorce, it was considered something to be ashamed of. And in the past it was an advantage held only by wealthy people . . . like the Grand Tour of Europe. No longer. Women and men are flocking to plastic surgeons to have nose bobs, eye bags removed, cheek tautened, mouth lines erased. I've had a go at it myself—five years ago a plastic surgeon made my eyes *seem* larger—a feat I'll tell you about in a later chapter. Today, few are so sensitive that they won't admit to having had cosmetic surgery. And it has become relatively less expensive.

When is the right time for cosmetic surgery? The minute you see that your face is beginning to wrinkle or sag. If you wait too long and have a lot of jowl and sag, a complete facial job might very well make you look so *different* that you'll be unhappy with the result. If you catch it early enough, there won't be that much contrast—and if you don't want to talk about it, friends will simply think you've been taking good care of yourself

SKIN—THE BIG WRAP

and look marvelous. It's better to get a nip here and a tuck there, in the early stages.

Personally, I think the skin peel will be the cosmetic lift of the future. One doctor I know describes the difference between a face lift and a skin peel in this way: "Pretend you have a sheet over your face. A face lift pulls at the sheet to make it taut. A skin peel gives you a new sheet." If you have a skin peel every three to five years, I believe you'll never have to have plastic surgery. A full face lift is major surgery and can require up to five hours on the operating table—and when it's all over, a skin peel is often recommended as an aftermath. You can have a face lift every five years, but why go through all that, including the trauma, when you can simplify the matter with face peels? The way they do peels today there is no scar, whereas plastic surgery on the face leaves scars in back of your ears and on your scalp.

If you've opted for a peel, be sure to find a doctor who specializes in peels. Ask to speak to, and if possible see patients on whom he has done a peel. You'll be assured he knows his craft if he explains that during the procedure, your kidneys will be flushed. This is most important for you to know. A skin peel is done with the use of phenyl and trichloroacetic acids. These are toxic and can be absorbed into the body, so while the peel is being done they attach an IV (intravenous) to an arm and flush the kidneys to prevent damage to these organs.

When done by a competent surgeon, a face peel is unbelievable. All the old layers of skin left over from the past fourteen-day sheddings are removed. A peel also removes wrinkles and superficial lines around the mouth. The aftermath is also much simpler than that of a face lift. With a face peel, you can return to work after seven or eight days, and in nine to ten days can apply make-up. For the first three days after the peel is done, you should stay in a convalescent hospital where there are nurses knowledgeable about post-peel care. At the very beginning, the skin is scabby, then looks red like a sunburn, for about three weeks, gradually lightening until your natural color has returned—usually in about twelve weeks.

To understand what a skin peel does, think about those leftovers of the fourteen-day skin shed. If they haven't been removed with proper skin care, that miniscule scaly matter gets into your pores and causes irritation. It's the same as though you'd applied daily makeup over the previous day's makeup all your life. At thirty, can you imagine how thick that buildup would be? That's what happens; your skin gets thick because you haven't exfoliated it, haven't removed the dry, flaking skin. That's why, as you grow older, skin is so leathery that you wrinkle when you smile. A skin peel corrects this, just by removing layers of old skin. If you've taken care of your skin from an early age, you may not need a peel.

Whatever you choose—lift or peel—please have consultations with at least three plastic surgeons. And I repeat, ask to see some of his former patients. You wouldn't buy a car without looking at it, would you? For any kind of surgery, even the peel, you should be in top nutritional condition. If you are, you'll fare better than a junk-food junkie. A good surgeon will suggest you have a complete physical first, including a series on blood. Don't consider a face lift while you are overweight. This is because if you reduce your weight later, your face will sag. A good plastic surgeon will explain all these things to you.

I stress that you have consultations with several plastic surgeons because they specialize like any other doctor. Some are experts on noses, some on chins or eyes, some on peels only. Plastic surgery can be dangerous territory, a fact Nanette Fabray knows well. When Nanette was twelve, an aunt decided to take charge of the girl's career and sent her off to have her nose done. In those days, they inserted a steel brace beneath the surface. Not long after, Nanette was caught in a blizzard and in such agonizing pain from the cold that they had to remove the steel. Subsequently, she's had to have her nose operated on again and again. Do all your checking beforehand, learn the doctors' track records, and which one specializes in what.

I stress another point. TELL YOUR DOCTOR THE TRUTH ABOUT YOUR PHYSICAL CONDITION. Totie Fields is a case in point, because she failed to admit she was diabetic. She consulted several plastic surgeons on the West Coast who refused surgery when they learned she had diabetes. So Totie went East, saw a doctor there, and purposely failed to mention her diabetic condition. Unaware of it, he gave her a face lift—which didn't take. The incisions did not heal and became infected. The medication then prescribed caused phlebitis in her leg, which eventually had to be amputated.

Jackie Gleason had a marvelous face lift. The results were so great that Jackie will talk about it to anyone who'll listen, and he is a prime example of what can be achieved.

It's a good idea to ask your doctor to do too little, rather than too much. Just as you'd ask your hairdresser not to cut your hair too short. If you have too much done in a face lift, you're more likely to look like someone else rather than yourself. Tell the doctor, "Leave a little nasal labial fold—I'd rather have lines from nose to mouth than have my upper lip look pulled up."

Joyce says that if you decide on a face lift, you can begin preparing yourself nutritionally two months beforehand. You'll heal much faster if you take a good B complex vitamin, plus vitamins A, C, and E. You will have less discoloration if you load up on 1,200 daily mgs. of calcium lactinate (maximum dosage) plus vitamin C.

One last thing about plastic surgery of any kind. (We'll get into plastic surgery of the body in Chapter 7, but what I'm about to say applies to that, too.) Please, please, if you've decided to improve your appearance in any way by surgery, do not fantasize that your life will miraculously change. Just because you look prettier, or younger, or sexier, doesn't necessarily mean you're now going to catch the man of your dreams, or that you'll be a smash at dinner parties. Your life will very probably go on exactly as before. I've known of so many women who go through the process of plastic surgery—which includes pain, puffiness, discoloration, and a term of withdrawal from society while healing—anticipating that everything will soon come up roses. If it turns out to be the same old grind, the same loneliness, the same problems, then they go through dreadful bouts of depression. If you choose plastic surgery, you should be doing it only for yourself, to smile a bit smugly when you look at your image in a mirror. About this, you should be honest with yourself.

This has been one fat chapter on the subject of your skin, but then you have more of it than anything else. Besides, it shows. You can hide a lot of defects, but with a beautiful skin, you're well on your way to being a charmer.

4
The Mane Thing

A friend of mine owns a beauty salon where the majority of customers are elderly women. She is driven slightly insane every time a poor old soul with nine hairs on her head totters in and says, "Make me look like Farrah Fawcett."

You can want hair like Farrah's, but hers is the texture that nature passes out to only one in a million. So regardless of your age, chances are you haven't a mane like hers. But, unless you are bald, you can have beautiful hair.

The first thing to learn about hair is that, like skin, it is made of protein. Under a microscope, a strand of hair is seen as link after link of protein. So in shampoos, conditioners, and rinses, as well as your diet, you should feed protein to your hair. Without it, hair will lose its luster, break, and ultimately part company with your head. (Incidentally, if you've bought liquid protein to take internally, don't throw it out after you read in Chapter 7 why you shouldn't swallow the stuff. Keep it and add a little to your rinse water, and your hair will absorb it, increasing in strength.)

The second thing to know about hair is that it is alive at the root, but once it grows out, it is a callus. This is why brushing is so important—you must spread the natural oils throughout the length of the hairs.

Thirdly, hair is almost always dirty. Every bit of city soot and country cobweb you walk through catches in your hair. In point of fact, hair is like a cobweb, snaring everything to which it's exposed. As a result, it is full of germs, and as I've already told you, should be kept away from your face, particularly if you have any blemishes.

As for the frequency of shampooing, that's a question women have been booting around for as long as I can remember. My best friend used to tell me I'd ruin my hair because I washed it so often. There is no proof that this is true. How often you shampoo depends entirely on you. Don't allow it to get greasy and don't let it dry out. It's a matter of body awareness, and no one knows your body better than yourself.

What makes hair oily or dry? Like skin, the oil factor is genetic, and it is the skin itself that affects the hair. The scalp is skin, and if it is oily, the hair becomes oily. An extremely oily condition signals that something is wrong. Too much oil coming from the system calls for a check on your nutritional balance; perhaps your intake of oils and fats should be reduced.

To keep a good balance, make certain you take the following vitamins. B complex in the proper ratio (1–2 tbsp. of brewers' yeast gives you this, but remember to start out with the smaller quantity and gradually increase), plus vitamins C, and A, the latter to prevent dryness and dandruff. Wheat germ and lecithin are great builders of the body of the hair, as are unsaturated oils. If your hair is dry, take an extra tablespoon of olive or safflower oil every day—in salad or the skin shake. If your hair is oily, cut down on oil intake. Iodine, iron, copper, and zinc should be balanced. To learn what you need, you can have an analysis made of your hair. It is a perfect barometer of the system; a few strands of hair will indicate the precise ratio of minerals in your body. Joyce does hair analysis, as do nutritionists and many doctors who practice preventive medicine. For a list of nutritionists, write to Albion Laboratories, 101 North Main Street, P. O. Box 750, Clearfield, Utah 84015.

PRE-SHAMPOO

The prologue of any shampoo is a good brushing while the hair is still dry. Always lean over and begin brushing at the nape of the neck, then work forward and along the sides of your head. If instead you brush from the top, standing in an upright position, the hair at the nape of your neck is neglected—and the back of your head is where you get the worst tangles.

Never use soiled brushes or combs. They should be cleaned at least once a week by soaking in warm soapy water. I always add a little ammonia to the water to assure cleanliness. Natural bristle brushes are far better than those made of nylon, which scratch the scalp. Natural bristles do not.

Now that you've brushed your hair, massage the scalp with your fingertips. Work in a circular motion, starting at the nape of the neck and moving up to the temples. This stimulates circulation, imperative for healthy hair.

If your hair is dry, now is the time for a good hot oil treatment. Using the best eye cream you have—or a moisturizer made with vegetable oils

THE MANE THING

(sesame, olive, or coconut oil)—put a dab on the palm of one hand and stroke your brush through it. With your head lowered (I'm quite aware you're spending a great deal of time upside down, but the blood is getting to your head, and that's good for you), start brushing, again at the back of your head. Use more cream if necessary and continue brushing until the hair is lightly coated. Massage again to make certain the oil has penetrated each strand. Then wrap around your head, Turk fashion, a towel that has been wrung out after soaking in hot water. Apply fresh hot towels for 15 or 20 minutes, then gently massage your scalp again before you shampoo.

If your hair is oily, here is a good "degreaser" to use before you shampoo. Beat the whites of two eggs, add plain yoghurt and a pinch of bicarbonate of soda, and work this mixture into your hair. This is like a facial for the hair; same thing—you're adding protein to protein.

Another conditioner for oily hair to be used before shampoo:

2 cups water
2 eggs
1 tsp. baking soda
Juice of half a lemon

Beat the eggs well with the lemon juice, then add baking soda and water. Pour over your hair and massage well into the scalp. Shampoo and rinse.

MAYONNAISE

Plain old kitchen mayonnaise is loaded with eggs, vegetable oil, and vinegar, and is great for any type of hair. Rub it in well, cover your hair with a plastic bag (Saran wrap will do), and sit under the dryer for 20 minutes while the heat makes the mayonnaise penetrate the hair strands. Or, if this is a day to pamper yourself, rub in the mayonnaise, cover with a shower cap and leave it on all day. Afterward, shampoo thoroughly—or someone will be tempted to toss a salad on your head.

THE SHAMPOO

Water temperature should be lukewarm, never too hot. No one's been able to improve on 98.6 for the human body. Finish with a cool rinse, which will close the scalp pores, thereby avoiding future lodging of dirt as well as catching cold.

A note about the way you shampoo. When I'm under stress my scalp tends to be itchy. This comes and goes, but when it's with me I'm always tempted to scratch my scalp when shampooing. The urge is to dig in with my nails, and I have to remind myself to take it easy. Massage of the scalp should be done briskly with finger*tips*. I'd suggest you warn your professional hairdresser, too—90 per cent of them wear witch-long nails, and plenty of them have given me some nasty digs. Any laceration is open to infection, and this is particularly dangerous when the shampoo will be followed by the application of chemicals, peroxide, a dye, a permanent solution, whatever. Preceding a bleach or tint, don't brush your scalp—confine brushing to the ends of your hair.

It's easier to shampoo in the shower than the sink or tub because you have a built-in waterfall that will more readily remove all shampoo.

After several rinsings in water, you should always apply a finishing rinse (recipes to come), then give it time to work while you bathe in the shower.

About drying your hair. The old-fashioned turkish towel is best. Hair dryers, whether professional or the type for home use, are just not good for your hair. They bake it. They also bake your face, which comes in for a lot of hot air. I'd suggest that if you frequent a beauty salon, you apply moisturizer to your face before you leave home. Or take some with you. I've seen Tina Louise smooth moisturizer over her face while she's actually under the dryer. The heat is good then, helping the moisturizer soak into your facial skin.

Whether at home or in a professional shop, remember that a dryer can burn your face and ears . . . ears in particular. How many times have you emerged from a dryer looking as though your ears were sunburned? Always tuck cotton balls around your face and ears, and never, never allow a metal clip to touch face, ears, or neck when you're under a dryer.

Few of us have time to allow our hair to dry naturally, which of course is the best method. If you must leave the house with a wet head, you may be asking for a cold. There's been a lot of recent research by the English, claiming there is no correlation between a wet head and catching cold; they say you're not going to catch cold unless your defenses are low. Regardless, unless you're in A-1 shape and look fabulous with a head of wet hair, I wouldn't suggest leaving the house that way.

Finally, when combing out wet hair, use a wide-toothed comb, and comb gently. I shouldn't have to warn you not to hack away at snarls—there's no faster way to break hundreds of hairs.

WHICH SHAMPOO

If you *must* buy a commercial shampoo, read the label first, and do not buy any shampoo containing alcohol, or color dyes which can be carcinogenic.

Do look for the ingredient of keratin protein, the structural protein of which hair and nails are made. It provides about 20 amino acids, whereas some of the collagen proteins contain only one or two amino acids. Keratin in a shampoo encourages thick, lustrous hair. If you can find a keratin powder, you can massage this onto your hair when wet, as it will mix with the natural oils of the hair. Or you can add a little keratin powder to your shampoo. Look for it at your drugstore.

EGG SHAMPOO
(FOR DRY HAIR AND/OR DANDRUFF)

- 1 pt. of water
- 1 egg
- 1 oz. rosemary

Brew the rosemary in water for 20 minutes, strain and cool. Add the egg to this tea and beat well. Massage into the scalp and hair, then rinse thoroughly.

BEER SHAMPOO

Mix beer with an equal amount of shampoo. Beer contains malt, hops, and yeast and is a good source of protein. It will do more for your hair than it does for your waistline.

DRY SHAMPOO

In show business, I often have to race from the television studio to some other kind of stage, or vice versa. I often find there isn't enough time to wash my hair, which requires an hour and a half to dry. I've found that good old Johnson & Johnson baby powder works wonders. I part my hair, a little bit at a time, and sprinkle the powder, rub it in thoroughly and then brush it out. It removes the oil, at least for a few hours until I have time for a regular shampoo. Of course, white powder is okay for blondes, but would appear rather dusty on dark hair. If yours is dark, use corn meal, whose coarse, granular texture can be brushed out easily. Rub it into your hair, wait five minutes and then brush it out. A dry shampoo comes in quite handy when you're desperate for time.

FINISHING RINSES

My hair is normal, neither dry nor oily, and if necessary I can go an entire week with my hair looking reasonably well. But a few years ago I noticed it quickly began to separate and look oily after two or three days. The only thing I'd been doing differently was using commercial cream rinses, those preparations touted to make your hair soft and fuller, and most particularly to straighten out tangles. So I stopped using them and my hair returned to normal. Now, of course, I use Joyce's herbal rinses. They don't contain any oily residue. I'll give you several, and you might experiment with all of them to learn which works best for you.

Joyce has told me that commercial cream hair rinses are made of the same formula as laundry rinses that soften clothes. The only difference is that the laundry rinses are a bit stronger and used with more water. Herbal rinses are better—you *know* what you're putting on your hair, you'll get fine results, and you don't have to remove most herbal rinses. You just leave them on as your hair dries. To any of the rinses Joyce recommends, you might add Panthenol in pill form (available at drugstores). Panthenol is a provitamin and is transformed into pantothenic acid in the body, even when applied externally. It's excellent not only for hair, but for skin. And while I'm on the subject, taken internally as a vitamin, Panthenol helps the intestinal flora to retain proper balance, aiding the problem of constipation.

Before I line up several natural hair rinses for you, I think it's important that you understand *why* you are using some of these ingredients. Vinegar and lemon juice are used because hair needs to be slightly acidic to maintain its health. (Soap is usually alkaline.) Eggs, too, are acidic, and also contain protein.

If you'd like to concoct a big batch of any of the following rinses so that you can keep it in the refrigerator, you might add agar-agar—which is a seaweed. (Unless you're a crossword puzzle buff you've probably never heard of agar-agar, and should look it up in "What's THAT?"—plus a whole batch of these rinse ingredients that may be new to you.) Agar-agar is loaded with vitamins and minerals and will add sheen to your hair. It has a jelling quality when heated in water, and the resultant consistency will make it easy for you to massage the rinse into your hair.

Here's how to do it. After making your rinse and straining it to remove the herbs, prepare the agar-agar jell by dissolving $\frac{1}{3}$ cup of agar-agar in 1 cup of water and boiling for 3 minutes. Then add the agar-agar with $\frac{1}{2}$ cup of cider vinegar to the rinse. Stir, heat to a simmer, then cool and keep refrigerated in a tightly closed jar. This makes a very concentrated rinse—you'll need to use only a little each time.

Most of the herbs used in the rinses are available in three forms—roots, leaves, or powder. Roots have the most power, and after being chopped or grated should be brewed an hour. Herbs in the form of leaves or powder should be tossed into the pot for the final few minutes—and at the very last minute, things recommended for essence.

I know it's confusing at first. When Joyce told me to use lemon grass on my hair, I said, "How am I going to carry home a bunch of grass? What is it? Turf from under a lemon tree?"

About sundry other weird-sounding herbs I said, "How can you measure a teaspoon of something that's twiggy?" Said Joyce, "It's *not* twiggy." And she was right. So relax, everything is easy, and Chapter 11 will answer all your questions.

To every rinse recipe Joyce and I give you, you can add a couple of things that will help your hair if it is very dry. You can use tannin, a natural astringent found in tea, which is good for dandruff as well as dry hair. Add ¼ cup of tea, and this will encourage moisture to leave but the oils to remain in the hair. Also, if your hair is very dry, you can add a little olive or safflower oil to the rinse. You will have to balance the amount of oil, depending on the condition of your hair. Start with a little at first, and you might add more later as you refine your formula. (Oil will rise in the jah, so be sure you shake before using.)

ROSEMARY RINSE

Rosemary is excellent for a rinse. Make a tea with 1 tsp. of rosemary to 2 cups of water. Boil for 10 minutes and steep, cool, then strain. If your hair tends to be oily add juice of half a lemon—or 2 tbs. of cider vinegar. With cool water, lightly rinse the rosemary from the hair before setting in your usual manner.

HERBAL RINSE

¼ oz. chopped quassia bark
¼ oz. chopped willow bark
¼ oz. chopped wild cherry bark

Simmer for one hour in a covered pot with 2 qts. of water, then add ½ oz. each of:

Lavendar flowers
Nettle
Rosemary
Rosebuds

Simmer gently 15 minutes, turn off the heat and allow the herbs to steep for a few hours, then strain. Mix into the brew 4 tbs. of aloe vera gel.

This rinse requires time to make, and I suggest you make up a batch and fill a few sterilized bottles. If you want to add agar-agar, add ⅓ cup and ½ cup of cider vinegar, as I've already explained. The cider vinegar will preserve the rinse for a while, but it's best if you refrigerate the bottles after they've been opened.

This is a concentrated rinse and you will need only a little on the palm of your hand. There is no need to rinse with water after application; the herbs will continue working on your hair. See Chapter 11 for availability of the herbs and flowers.

HERBAL RINSE FOR OILY HAIR

    1 qt. of water
    ¼ oz. of burdock root

Simmer this brew for one hour, then add ¼ oz. each:

    Lemon grass
    Nettle
    Onion leaves (either chopped natural leaves, or those purchased from your grocer's spice shelf)
    Peach leaves
    Rosemary
    Southernwood
    Yarrow flowers

Simmer these for 10 minutes, then store and use as the preceding herbal rinse.

HERBAL RINSE FOR DRY HAIR

    1 qt. of water
    ¼ oz. burdock root
    ¼ oz. comfrey root
    ¼ oz. wild cherry bark
    ¼ oz. camomile

Simmer for one hour, then add ½ oz. of each of the following:

    Clover
    Elder flowers
    Papaya leaves
    Peach leaves
    Rosemary

Brew these for 15 minutes and prepare as preceding rinses.

HAIR LOSS

Women tend to panic when they notice their hair is falling out. Men aren't exactly ecstatic at the prospect of baldness, but it seems to me they're a lot calmer about it than women, perhaps because they've learned to live with the anticipation of a receding hairline. (If castrated at puberty, men will not go bald. I guess the anticipation of a receding hairline is easier for them to live with.)

I joined the panic club when I discovered a bald spot near the hairline at the center of my forehead. It was only the size of a nickel, but I remember staring at it in horror. Then I remembered my acting role at the time required a wig, and they had supplied me with exceptionally tight wigs. When the role ceased, so did the wigs, and new hair eventually grew into the spot. Luckily, the hair follicles hadn't been destroyed. But for a long time I couldn't wear a center part. Pressure resulting from anything too tight on your head—even a fall—will cause hair loss. So, too, will stress and nutritional deficiency.

Research with animals has shown that their coats are restored with the use of natural linseed oil. *Not* the kind you buy at a paint store, but linseed oil purchased at a pharmacy. It is nature's product, made from flax seed. You might well benefit by massaging linseed oil on areas of your scalp where hair is thinning. Or adding 1 tablespoon of linseed oil to your daily diet.

Or try the following as a finishing rinse after your shampoo.

RINSE FOR FALLING HAIR

    1 qt. of water
    ¼ oz. burdock root
    ¼ oz. comfrey root
    ¼ oz. willow bark
Simmer for one hour, then add and simmer for 10 minutes:
    ½ oz. basil
    ½ oz. camomile
    ½ oz. clover
Cool and strain.

THE SUN AND YOUR HAIR

No need to tell you the sun plays havoc with hair. It dries it, breaks it, bleaches it, burns it, kills it.

To protect your hair, Joyce suggests using the same sun block you apply to your skin. Be sure the block contains PABA (paramino-benzoic acid), which is one of the B vitamins. This is particularly essential for redheads and fair-haired people, who have a tendency to be sensitive to the sun's rays. (Don't I know it!) Do not buy any product whose label states it may discolor bleached or tinted hair.

If you're going to the beach and don't want to goop up your hair with a sun block, cover your head with a hat or scarf. In the privacy of your own garden or patio, incidentally, you might protect your hair and condition it at the same time with an application of mayonnaise.

My final warning is about chlorine. If, after you've been swimming in a pool, you open your eyes the next morning to discover they're flaming red, you can imagine what chlorine does to hair. My own turns an interesting shade of green. I don't know what it does to yours, but I strongly suggest that if you've allowed chlorine to run through your hair, you correct it as soon as possible with a shampoo and a conditioner. At the very least, rinse your hair in the shower and avoid drying it in the sun.

HAIR COLOR

"Does she or doesn't she?" is old hat. No one cares any more if you change the color of your hair. I know many women who've tinted their hair for so many years that they haven't the least idea whether or not they've begun to turn gray. There hasn't been an opportunity to find out.

On the subject of gray hair, I'd like to put in a pitch for it. I think it looks smashing on the majority of women lucky enough to sprout it. My Aunt June has salt-and-pepper hair down to her waist, and looks fabulous. If we think gray or silver hair on a man is attractive, why not on you? If you've begun turning gray, it is a natural change and goes with your complexion, and I think you should strongly consider letting nature take its course.

If you do want to change color, think about shades other than blonde. I don't believe blondes have more fun than anybody, and you have a wide range of shades to choose from. (Just don't have it dyed black. Black-black hair—unless natural, as with orientals—always looks as though a woman has been doused with a bucketful of lacquer.)

A word about recent warnings that hair dyes may be carcinogenic. This refers to *dyes,* for red, black, and brown hair—not the one-step tints. It seems women are not paying attention to the likelihood that hair dyes can cause cancer, and the alert about hair dyes is being largely ignored. The sensible answer, if you want to change hair color in the range of darker shades, is to use a natural product, and I suggest henna.

HENNA

Henna has been used effectively and safely since the time of the ancient Egyptians. There are two kinds—neutral and red. The neutral henna does not color the hair, but thickens it and brings out natural highlights. It is excellent for making fine and/or sparse hair look and feel thicker. It's a great conditioner, and you can feel the difference immediately after washing your hair. For this reason, I wouldn't touch it with a ten-foot pole; my hair is already too thick to control easily

Then there's red henna, which will give any shade of brown hair lovely red highlights. My best friend has brown hair and uses red henna, and looks sensational—particularly in sunlight. The stronger your mixture, the redder your hair, so be cautious the first few times you use it. Both the neutral and red henna coat the hair, which makes it hold moisture longer, so be advised that if you use henna much more time will be required to dry your hair.

For red hair, Joyce suggests that you slowly stir 2 cups of red henna powder into 1 cup of tepid water and make a paste thick enough so that it won't drip from the scalp and hair. You may further improve a henna dye by adding 1 tsp. of pure cider vinegar and ½ tsp. of Golden Seal (see Chapter 11) in powder form. Heat the mixture slowly in a double boiler, and when it's near to a boil, keep it on the flame for a few minutes. Then remove from the fire and steep for an hour. Finally, reheat the mixture to body temperature and massage well into the hair. Tie a scarf over your head while the henna is working and leave it on for at least seven hours. Then rinse with warm water, and apply a little oil to the scalp and hair.

For a red hair rinse, simmer ½ oz. of henna in 1 qt. of water for 20 minutes. Rinse this through the hair several times, then rinse with water 3 times. The final rinse should be 1 oz. of cider vinegar mixed in 8 oz. of water. Be careful if your hair is naturally gray or white, as the color of red henna accumulates.

For a reddish-brown color, use ½ oz. of red henna to ½ oz. of camomile.

To add a warm chestnut color to fading brown hair, combine ¼ oz. of red henna to ¾ oz. of camomile.

If you live in the country, pick walnuts or pecans and boil the shells. Joyce's aunt in Texas has done this for years, using the brew as a rinse. It gives hair a lovely shade of brown; the longer you brew the nut shells, the darker the shade. This stains the hair, and will not come off. Thus, I suggest you wear rubber gloves while applying it, and apply cold cream around the hairline and neck so that it won't stain your skin. If it does, don't panic or try to remove it with alcohol. Henna stays on hair, but with the help of your natural oils will disappear from skin in a couple of days.

If you opt for blond hair, here is a natural lightener.

HAIR LIGHTENER

Simmer slowly for 1 hour 8 oz. of camomile in ½ pt. of water. Strain, and apply with cotton pads. Leave on the hair for 30 minutes, rinse with the juice of a lemon in water, and for the final rinse use clear water. Repeat application may be necessary.

BLOND TONER

Simmer for 30 minutes ¼ cup of camomile in 1 pt. of water. Cool and add 1 tsp. of lemon juice. Strain, then rinse through hair several times before final rinse with clear water.

WIGS

If you wear a wig or fall, be sure to remove it as often as possible to allow air to reach your head. Wigs do make the scalp perspire. Don't wear a wig that's too tight; this not only prevents the scalp from being aerated, but may rub the scalp and damage hair follicles—as I've already discovered. If your head has been shaved for surgery, it is most important that your wig not be too tight.

To make a wig look less wiggy, pull out about an inch of your own hair all around the hairline, and comb it carefully into the hairs of the wig. Dolly Parton does this with those Nashville numbers she wears. There's nothing worse than a wig that is obviously a wig. I've seen women, in public, pull one side open and poke a finger in there to scratch. Or worse, grab their wig as though it were a hat, and rock it back and forth. I'm sure their thoughts are a mile off and they don't realize how ridiculous they look. If you wear a wig, *remember* you're wearing it.

HAIR STYLE

The way you wear your hair can't actually change your facial shape, but it can certainly make it *look* different. If you have a square jaw, wear your hair long enough that it can partially cover that part of your face. If your face is longish, wear a short bob with hair full at the sides. If your face is thin, pull the hair away from it at the side, then fluff it out a bit. If your forehead is short and you don't want the bad hairline to show, wear bangs started well back on the head.

It's really quite simple; just apply the opposite of the fault. And remember, hair is a frame for the face and a frame should never overwhelm its picture. Crowning glory it may be, but don't wear it in such a cloud that your face peeps out like a postage stamp. I used to wear my hair hanging close to my face, hoping it would visually cut off half of my cheeks. I now realize I look much more attractive if I pull it away from my face instead.

Hair is always thicker on one side than the other. Finding out which side is simple; just part your hair in the center and feel each side. We're different all over our bodies, one side from the other. This difference stems from the very first time our original cell divided in half. So we have one foot slightly larger, one hand, one breast, and each side of our face is different. It's said that Claudette Colbert is the only mortal known to man with a completely symmetrical face. When you know which side of your hair is the thicker, part it on that side, giving the thinner side more hair to play with.

HAIR IN PHOTOGRAPHY

If you plan having your photograph taken, don't get a new hairdo the day before. Forever after, you'll look at the photograph and tell yourself, "That's not what I looked like." My sister got a new hairdo for her wedding portrait, in which she looks no more like herself than the man in the moon. When actresses plan a portfolio they start a month ahead, practicing hairdos and learning which is the most attractive for them. If you decide on a haircut, have it done two months before the photograph to allow time for growth and change in the event you dislike the cut. And don't wear your hair so that it looks like cement. The more natural and soft the look, the better. In fact, if your photographer has a fan in his studio, have him use it to blow your hair just a bit during the session. This gives a free, airy look to the photo and relieves rigidity.

LONG OR SHORT?

There's an old saw that says older women should not wear their hair long, that the swinging mane is strictly for the young. I think this is true in general, but I know quite a few women of middle age who wear it long and look attractive. They can carry it off because of their personalities. Colleen Dewhurst is one; she's such an earth mother type that it works well for her. Another is Betty Garrett Parks, who switched from "All in the Family" to "Laverne and Shirley." Betty doesn't always let it hang loose; sometimes she wraps it into a bun or wears it in a pony tail. When Betty did a one-woman stage show she let her hair down while playing a bride, then swept it up for other moments in her show. An advantage of long hair is that you can do so many things with it. Then there's my idol, Ruth Gordon. We're so accustomed to this perky little lady in her 80s with long hair that I doubt we'd recognize her in a short haircut. Ruth sometimes rolls it up—or wears a wig for a role. But she's an individualist; sometimes she braids it, sometimes she even puts it up and wears a man's hat. Individualism is the key word on the question of age-related long or short hair. If an older woman can get away with it and make it an advantage, then good for her.

But in general, the age at which a woman should cease wearing long hair comes on the day when she looks in a mirror and decides her face needs an uplift. When the lines begin going down and the chin seems lower than ever before, long hair only promotes the downward trend. Short hair will visually lift the face.

Another point about long hair is your personal thermostat. Mine is on a naturally high setting, and I begin to perspire in the slightest warm weather. Some people, the desert-rat type, thrive on heat, and others are cold regardless of room temperature. My husband, Bill, has an interesting theory about this difference. He thinks it might be genetic, going back for centuries. His ancestors come from the hot plains of Israel, and the hotter the weather, the happier is Bill. My forebears were Scandinavian and Scottish, and I love winter weather.

Relating hair to this, mine is very thick, and it's like wearing a fur coat on my head. Great hanging down my neck when it's cold, but when it's hot I'm uncomfortable all over. The neck is almost like a pulse point, as when you run cold water over your wrists to cool off. Cooling off your neck will do wonders in summer, or when you're going to go out dancing and know you'll be warm—or appearing in court and know you'll be nervous, or if you're in menopause and suffering hot flashes. Allowing air to reach your neck is the answer—just sweep it up, or tie a ribbon around it in a ponytail. *Not* a rubber band—which breaks the hairs.

Do men prefer women with long hair or short hair? Many men say they like long hair, but if hair is attractive I don't believe it makes that much difference. A woman with a short and sassy cut can be just as alluring as one with long, flowing hair.

If you want your tresses to charm men out of their wits, hair must be clean—and it should have a nice aroma. If you smoke, or if you work in a place where others smoke, you should wash your hair every single day with a good mild shampoo. Hair shouldn't look "done." It's a turnoff for a man when he gets the urge to run his hands through your hair, and then hesitates because he's afraid he might ruin the set. Hair should look soft, not like concrete.

Very few girls are cute and saucy enough to carry off a totally boyish cut. There's a way of wearing your hair short without looking as though you posed for a Dutch Cleanser ad. Yet a lot of professionals do these boyish cuts. Some women can get away with it, like Mia Farrow with those enormous eyes. But just because she wears a short cut well, don't be certain that you can. Do you want a man to fall in love with you—or feel compelled to take you home and give you a good meal? Femininity is the answer for most of us—I don't know what's attractive about looking as though you've just been released from a concentration camp. You might wear your hair short if: (1) you have a long face, or (2) it's stringy, thin, or baby fine. A good short cut can make hair look much fuller.

But not too short, unless you want somebody to hail you with, "Hey sailor, when did you get into town?"

CUTS

Please, when a new cut is "in" don't race off to the barber chair or beauty salon. Don't let anybody talk you into it, including beauticians, just because it's "in style." I've seen women streaming out of a Beverly Hills shop, all looking as though they'd just come off an assembly line. The same, identical heads. Some looked great, some looked just awful, as though they were wearing a bowl on their heads. Maybe the original cut was great for a young oriental model (who'd probably look good in any hairdo) —but what's best for *your* face, *your* age, *your* life?

The same advice goes for long-hair styles. So many women are trying to look like Farrah Fawcett, but most of them never quite get the hang of it and succeed only in looking as though they're wearing a sausage at each side of the face. It also makes me think they have no sense of style, that they're just copycats, and can't think of anything right for themselves.

Before you let anyone cut your hair, before you take that picture of Cheryl Tiegs or Cher from a magazine to your beautician, *think* if it's right for your face and your age. Know that it's a bad cut if it looks good at the shop, but you can't reproduce the style at home. Who has the time or money to go to a beauty salon three times a week? It's a bad cut for you if you can't handle it by yourself in the interim.

You should have your hair cut when it's too long to retain its style. Or when long, thick hair is so stubborn it won't hold curl. In this case, I suggest it be thinned, and its style changed to one more layered. Layering doesn't have to show; it can be cut underneath so that it looks the same length but the hairs underneath are a couple of inches shorter. In my own case, wearing it long and hanging as I do most of the time, I have it trimmed once every six to eight weeks because this makes it look healthier. It's never been proven that cutting per se is good for hair, although some experts say it stimulates growth. It's good to have it cut occasionally simply to remove unhealthy ends. I'd like to let mine grow to my waist, but it's not possible because the ends of the hair are split or broken off and look so scraggly that I have to get it trimmed.

Cutting makes hair look fuller. I've seen girls with hair to their waist, with straggly ends that have begun to thin out a whole twelve inches from the bottom. I wonder why they're proud of its length when, if they had a foot or so cut off, it would look much fuller at the ends.

Hairs grow approximately one-quarter inch each month, but this is average. Some grow faster than others, so that after a few weeks the lengths are different.

(A macabre little note here, while I'm holding forth on hair. Did you know that hair—and nails—continue growing for about two weeks after death?)

Once you've decided whether you prefer your hair cut while dry or wet (it'll be more even when cut wet), be sure to check out any new operator. If they've been trained to cut one way, there's no use arguing with them. And know that when hair dries, it's considerably shorter than when wet. So if you're having a wet cut, caution the wielder of shears not to cut it too short.

I won't go into the subject of setting hair. If you set your own, you already have your procedure, I'm sure, whether with rollers with inside brush, or smooth plastic rollers. But there's one tip I can give you if you have very long hair. As a naturally wavy long-hair myself, I know you can use large orange juice cans (empty, of course), which are larger than the largest roller I've been able to find. One on each side of your head all day may make you look like a plugged-in Martian, but when you go out at night, your hair will be smooth and straight with a slight curl only at the ends.

One other tip, an important one—pry open bobby pins with your fingers, *not* your teeth. My dentist told me he's seen more front teeth damaged from bobby pins than he can shake a drill at.

A final plea. Please don't leave the privacy of your home with hair up in curlers. Done up in wire or plastic or fruit cans, even Miss Universe would look like a leftover from a rummage sale.

5
The Eyes Have It

In prose and poetry, eyes have been given more attention than any other feature of the body. They are the windows of the soul, they have seen the glory, and they send out tongues of love. You are asked to keep one peeled; also to drink to somebody with thine eyes. In them are fire, mud, stars, dreams, pearls, flash, sparkle, and fire. Young maidens have quiet eyes, the night has a thousand of them, and they're not open before marriage. Some things are sights for sore eyes (which can even be jaundiced), and in a bilious mood, Hart Crane described eyes as unwashed platters.

For the purpose of my book, I prefer Galsworthy's line, "One's eyes are what one is." He added, "One's mouth is what one becomes"—which is a good thought to grab the next time you are looking grumpy.

This reminds me of a story about Abe Lincoln. After he had interviewed a man for a government post, an aide remarked that the applicant seemed fit for the job.

"I don't like his face," said Lincoln.

"But, sir, the man can't control the look of his face!"

"I disagree," said old Abe. "By the time any man is thirty, he is totally responsible for his face."

You might tack that one on your bathroom mirror.

Your eyes show what you are, mentally, spiritually, and physically. They have an importance even beyond their blessing of sight, and it goes without saying that you should take care of them, primarily by having an annual checkup by an opthamologist or optometrist. A good specialist will not fail to check your eyes thoroughly, including tests for glaucoma. This disease can lead quickly to total blindness if undetected, and the bad news about glaucoma is that the type *without* symptoms of pain is the more dangerous. Only your eye doctor can discover its presence . . . along with other illnesses signaled by the eyes.

Without a doctor's help, you can care for your eyes in many ways. A simple rule is never to rub them, but if you must, use the backs of your hands rather than your fingers, which are usually soiled, not to mention the germs on your fingertips.

If a foreign object gets into your eye, it's particularly important not to rub it; this might well create a scratch on the surface of the eye. I know of three ways to remove an offending particle. (1) Bathe the eye with warm water, using an eye cup. Place the cup over your eye, tilt your head backward, then open and close the eye while it is exposed to the water. (2) Gently pull your upper eyelid over the lower lid, then roll your eye in all directions. This should dislodge the object. (3) With extreme care, hold the cotton end of a Q-Tip on your upper eyelid and fold the lid upward and over it. This bares the eye, enabling you to locate the foreign particle.

Never touch the eyes themselves with anything. If all the foregoing methods fail, make a quick trip to your doctor and have him remove the object.

When smoothing cream or oil around your eyes, use a circular motion outward under the brow, then inward under the eyes. The reverse direction pulls the skin beneath the eyes toward the temple and will break down this delicate tissue. Result: bags and wrinkles.

Never apply vinegar or any solution containing alcohol near your eyes. This includes perfume, which has an alcoholic content, and face masks, some of which contain alcohol and can be drying.

Make certain your eye cream does not contain mineral oil, which interferes with the absorption of vitamin A. You can improve effectiveness of eye cream by adding to it the oil squeezed from a vitamin E capsule.

Take vitamins A and C, both found in carrots, which will help prevent night blindness. My mother is night blind, and I have to keep reminding her to eat carrots—which is a mother-daughter switch.

Joyce reminds us that if you have puffs beneath your eyes, or dark circles, it's usually a sign you're deficient in vitamin C, which is necessary for the proper formation of collagen. Vitamin C is rapidly depleted by smoking. So cut that down, or *out*. Puffiness might also indicate that your salt intake is too high; try to avoid salt. Or the cause might be an accumulation of toxins in the liver. Your eyes will vastly improve, in themselves as well as the skin surrounding them, if you go on periodic one-to-three-day fasts, drinking the fasting broth discussed in Chapter 2. This detoxifies the liver, an organ that has a strong affect on appearance of both skin and eyes.

As an external treatment for dark circles or puffiness, use a potato compress once a day. Shred potatoes, wrap them in a moistened handkerchief or cheesecloth, and apply lightly beneath your eyes while you relax for 20 minutes. Or use cucumber slices applied in the same manner. Cucumbers have a soothing effect as well as helping to correct dark circles. A third treatment is a damp tea bag used in the same way.

If your eyes are tired from strain or have been exposed to too much sunlight, Joyce suggests that you make a soothing eye lotion by boiling 2 tsps. of cut celandine herb (see Chapter 11)—including the flowers if available—in 1 pt. of water. When cooled, add 1 part of this herb brew to 1 part of raw milk, and bathe your eyes with the solution.

Another brew can be made from an herb called eyebright. Add 1 tsp. of eyebright to 1 pt. of boiling water, then steep for 15 minutes. Cool, and apply with cotton pads soaked in the solution.

Eyes will feel rested after the use of a compress made with potatoes, cucumbers, or tea bags. Never apply these substances directly to the eye; always wrap them in fine cheesecloth or a clean handkerchief.

If your eyes are like mine, after sixty seconds of crying, they are red and puffy messes. You can correct this by wrapping a couple of ice cubes in a wash cloth, then applying them to your eyes while lying down for about five minutes.

I trust you're not sitting there with a black eye, but if so, I'm not there to ask any nosy questions. The best application for a shiner is ice or something cool, as soon as possible, to prevent swelling and the accumulation of blood. Afterward, treat it (or them) with compresses of potato or cucumber. Or the old prescription of a steak—it's not the *steak* that heals, but the enzymes in the steak. Potatoes are cheaper.

(I know how you feel. A few months ago I cracked my nose in my Kung Fu class and had two black eyes three days later. Not only that, I made a movie called *Intimate Strangers* dealing with battered wives, and when in makeup for my role my face was blue and yellow. It was interesting the way people avoided me. Those who didn't know about the movie seemed acutely embarrassed when talking with me, and looked everywhere but *at* my face. People seem to automatically assume you've been socked by your husband and feel uncomfortable and sorry for you.)

Again, if your eyes are tired, Joyce says that if you rub the palms of your hands together for a few minutes (as though drying your hands under one of those damned hot-air blowers in public rest rooms) and then cup them over your open eyes, the energy in your hands will radiate to the eyes.

To strengthen your eye muscles, here's a simple exercise. Keeping your head straight ahead and motionless, look as far to the left as possible, then right, then up, then down. There isn't a muscle in your body that won't improve with exercise.

Sun may be great to provide you with vitamin D (which along with A helps assimilate your calcium), but too much of it is rotten for your eyes. They burn much the same way as your skin, so protect them with sunglasses. You'll not only avoid burning your eyeballs, but you won't squint—and squinting is a dandy way to make wrinkles. Blue eyes, incidentally, are more sensitive to sunlight; you might have noticed that blue-eyed people squint more than others.

Sunglasses in dark shades of brown, green, or gray are best for your eyes. Yellow lenses are the worst because they intensify the brightness, so avoid them. Wear sunglasses when driving or when exposed to any bright light, as well as sunlight. I know several women who won't wear sunglasses because of the white circles left around the eyes where they've been covered. Makeup can camouflage these circles, but the simplest answer is to wear a hat, thereby protecting your whole face while you're at it.

GLASSES

Dorothy Parker did us a disservice when she wrote, "Men seldom make passes at girls who wear glasses." Personally, I prefer them to the use of contact lenses because I think eyeglasses can be so attractive.

The shape of the frame is important, of course. With my round face, I need wider frames to make my face look narrow. If your face is narrow, you should choose narrow glasses. Don't wear frames that are overly large—despite current styles. They can look as though *they* are taking you down the street. Or too small—the tiny ones look like two polka dots held together by wire. Do try on all sorts of shapes and find one that looks best for you. Bill and I finally got his mother to change her frames. We knew she needed something new when our wedding pictures came back from the photographer. Mrs. Rader's glasses had aluminum frames, and the light from flash bulbs bounced off them so that only frames were visible, no eyes. Now she has lightweight plastic frames, much larger, that open her face and give a more youthful look. They're tinted slightly with a rose color, which reflects well on her cheeks. She's a lovely woman, and now her new glasses allow everyone to see her beauty.

If you wear glasses, be very particular about the makeup that shows beneath them. Remember that your skin is magnified by the glass, and a heavy makeup can come off as overdone when seen through glasses.

Individuality is a keystone of beauty. Peter Falk and Sandy Duncan each have only one good eye—and who cares? They are as attractive as they ever were. Both Barbra Streisand and Karen Black have one eye that is slightly off center, but I haven't heard anyone complaining that either lacks charisma.

If you like the idea of contact lenses, there's a wonderful advantage to them because you can have the fun of changing eye color. When I had a movie role of a Jewish girl in *Hey, I'm Alive,* I had my hair dyed brown and wore brown contact lenses over my blue eyes. It's fascinating to be able to change your appearance like that—except that I had to cry in most of my scenes, and the brown lenses kept sloshing around and showing the rims of my blue eyes. Anyway, if you have light-colored eyes, you can get lenses to make them look blue, lavendar, gray, or green. You can do fabulous cosmetic things with the color of contact lenses. Don't be afraid to wear them, if your eye doctor approves—they're really quite easy to insert, and that statement comes from one of the world's biggest chickens, me. They're now made of a soft material that makes them more comfortable than the old-fashioned rigid ones. An additional plus—bifocal contact lenses don't *look* like bifocals.

PLASTIC SURGERY

Makeup can change the appearance of your eyes, but plastic surgery can actually change them. I know, because I've had it done. Five years ago, I had a manager who noticed my every flaw, and flapped over each like a mother hen. Every time I'd reach for bread, she'd slap my hand and say, "Fat!" One day when she was looking at still photographs of me she said, "You know, Sally, you have big eyes, but they don't look as big as they are because of this fatty fold on your upper eyelids. Maybe you ought to have those folds removed."

The surgeon I chose assured me the change would be so slight that no one would notice, but it *would* give me a more open-eyed look. He was right on both counts. The surgery was done in his office, after which he plopped dark glasses on me and sent me home for a couple of days of recouping. About a week later, stitches removed, I could use a light makeup base, wear tinted sunglasses and go out in public. It was painless, there was no scar, and since then on camera my eyes look as large and open as they really are.

Most women think of plastic surgery for fifty-year-olds; I had mine done when I was twenty-four. There are many ways in which eyes can be improved by cosmetic surgery—removal of bags beneath them, for example—and if you have a problem in this area you might think about consulting a few surgeons.

I've said I had no scar. That's not quite true. There was a hairline thin scar at first, but it quickly disappeared. If you've had plastic surgery relating to your eyes and have a scar, apply a little makeup base to your eyelids and then powder them lightly before applying shadow. Be sure you use a dark shadow, and blend it carefully over the scar.

EYEBROWS

Eyebrows most definitely affect the appearance of your eyes. In a way, they are a frame, so remember that the frame should never overwhelm the painting. If you have Joan Crawford eyebrows—heavy, heavy—they make your eyes look small, and you should pluck the unwanted hairs. There's a way to figure how to shape them. You measure three dimensions— (1) width of each eye, (2) distance from outer corner of eyes to temple, and (3) the width between your eyes. There should be a proper balance there; no one space should be wider than the others. If you find the space between your eyebrows is too narrow, the hairs are growing too close together. Pluck them so that they begin above the inner corner of the eye. To learn where they should stop at the outer sides, place a pencil at the side of your nose, extending it past the outer edge of the eye to the brow. This is the point at which the eyebrow should cease. If it extends beyond this point, pluck unwanted hairs; if it does not reach that far, extend it with a soft pencil.

For instructions on how to tweeze, plus more information about eyebrows, see page 118 in Chapter 6.

Does the color of your eyebrows match your hair? It isn't unusual for a difference in shade—many dark and light-haired men have red facial hair. My own eyebrows are much darker than my hair, and it bothered me when I was younger. My grandmother, a religious woman who believed all things should be totally natural, used to suspect I was bleaching my hair. I'd come home from college and she'd rub my eyebrows with her thumb and say, "Are you using an eyebrow pencil?" Silly question. My eyebrows were thick and very dark—too thick and too dark. She couldn't understand why, when my hair was blonde. "Well then, you must be bleaching your hair."

"Oh, Nanny, please stop."

Then I came to Hollywood and learned that eyebrows can be bleached.

They told me that the combination of light hair and dark eyebrows tends to make the eye appear heavy and closed.

To bleach, apply a little oil bleach on your eyebrows from 5–7 minutes —or use some Arctic Blonde toner. If your eyebrow hairs tend toward red, use toner to lighten them; this is better than straight bleach. A toner such as Arctic Blonde will lighten without turning them red. Remove any application with cool water on a towel, and don't rub too hard.

For a nice, open-eyed look, train the eyebrow hairs upward, rather than lying horizontally on the brow. Sophia Loren does this; so does Mary Tyler Moore. Comb them upward and trim any that stand too high above the horizontal line you want to create. To make them stay up, apply a little hair spray on your eyebrow brush and brush upward. Or, wet a finger, rub it on soap, then use that finger to brush brows upward.

If your eyebrows are sparse, encourage growth by rubbing them with a little castor oil every night. Or if you can't stomach castor oil, massage them with linseed oil. (Again, *natural* linseed oil—not the kind at the paint store.) And if they're sparse, or you have none at all, for heaven's sake please do not pencil them on by drawing one long line. Most unattractive. Instead, make short, hairlike strokes with the sharp point of your pencil, and sketch yourself natural-looking eyebrows.

6
Let's Make Up

Except for the very end of this chapter, which will be all about makeup when posing for photography—and that's my bag—I'm going to turn this one over to Joyce Virtue. Makeup is *her* bag. She is one of the top experts in the business, trusted by scores of actresses to make them even more beautiful than they are. Some of the famous faces Joyce makes up . . . Bea Arthur, Mary Tyler Moore, Tina Louise, Luci Arnaz, Cloris Leachman, Elke Sommers, Anna Maria Alberghetti, Carole White, Fannie Flagg, Joan Rivers. Actors come under her talented hands, too . . . Andy Williams, George Hamilton, John Denver are a few examples.

Makeup means making up for what isn't there, and enhancing what *is* there. If you've been paying attention, your skin is very possibly flawless now, and you can go anywhere without makeup. Can, but probably don't want to, because miracles are wrought by makeup . . . eyes intensified, color heightened, flaws camouflaged, good features enhanced.

I've never seen a truly ugly woman—every one of us has at least one feature that can be improved . . . eyes, nose, lips, cheeks, hair.

Learn the rule that applies to everyone, regardless of age. THE BEST MAKEUP JOB LOOKS AS THOUGH YOU'RE NOT WEARING ANY. Too much worsens the entire picture.

The occasion sets the amount. Surely, you're not going to swing around a golf course with eyelids caked in eyeshadow—and perspiration. Or attend Easter Sunday services wearing eyeliner like Cleopatra's. For sports, you're best off with lipstick, moisturizer, and a makeup base on top of your sun block. You need all the protection you can get from sunlight.

For your job, whatever it may be, keep makeup to a prudent whisper—you're supposed to be working, not looking for Mr. Goodbar.

If you're going dancing or have a dinner date, go to the end of the gamut, but keep in mind that you'd like your escort to compliment you on how beautiful you look, not comment on your interesting makeup job.

Weather also dictates the amount of makeup. Summer calls for a natural look, as sunlight magnifies makeup. Before leaving home, always check if you've done too much by taking a mirror (and your face) into a natural light, sunlight if possible. A worthwhile investment is one of the new mirrors that show your face in three kinds of light—daytime, office, and evening.

Be particularly careful to blend your foundation at the line of demarcation from chin to neck, an area often neglected by many women.

Winter's gray days demand more moisturizer, and more color on your face. In autumn, if you're losing a summer tan, mix your darker summer and lighter winter bases together and gradually lighten the tone as the weeks go by.

Makeup takes time. You shouldn't just slap it on and tear out of the house. Sally uses up 40 minutes for a full makeup, and so is incredulous at my own speed. But I have to look my best at all hours because I'm in the *business* of applying makeup, and by now I have my morning routine down to 30 minutes. Practice not only makes perfect, but lessens the time required. In that half hour—following my exercises—I set my hair, apply my daily facial mask of oatmeal, honey, and almond meal, and leave this on while I shower and shave my legs. I finish with a cold shower, rinsing off the facial, and after toweling, "dry brush" my face with a dry towel to increase circulation. Then I apply moisturizer, and a full makeup.

About cosmetics. They all have the same basic ingredients, except that those I recommend are made with vegetable oil or lanolin (the latter only for extremely dry skin) and never mineral oil. They usually contain glycerine and petroleum, of which Vaseline is a derivative. **Musk and** turtle oil, despite claims made for them, have no advantage over **lanolin**. Musk oil is used for perfume only. Turtle oil must always be cut or **emulsified** with lanolin. But why use turtle oil when vegetable oil is so **much better**?

You can be an artist with a makeup brush. The best **brushes are** made of sable, and are available at any art supply store. The advised **width is** $1\frac{1}{2}''$ for powder, and one a little wider for blush on. Powder **puffs are** not recommended; they not only become soiled, but produce **a caked look**. Other than your fingers, sable brushes and cotton balls are **the only tools** you need for makeup application, plus a lip brush—the best applicator for lipstick and gloss—and a soft-lead eye pencil.

THE 15 MINUTE MAKEUP

Before you begin, cleanse your face and apply a moisturizer, which is needed by oily skin as well as dry. If extremely oily, use a cotton ball to apply an astringent before moisturizer to remove all oil. A fine moisturizer is mineral water (such as Evian or Perrier). Mineral waters are good for both keeping moisture under the skin and for setting makeup. Just spray them on.

Try to work in a north light, the light used by painters because of its clarity. And as you work, remember that there should be a balance between the eyes, cheeks, and lips. Women often make up their eyes, put on a blush powder, and forget to do anything about their lips. This makes their eyes look overdone. Balance is important.

1. Use a cover up to lighten any discolorations or dark circles.

2. Use a base on the eyelids, from eyelashes all the way to the eyebrow. (Foundation is not recommended here because it is so oily that eye makeup won't adhere.) When buying your base, ask for a "base for eyelids." These are manufactured by cosmetic companies under various names.

3. Apply foundation by patting it on with your fingertips. (If you rub it, it will streak.) Pat it on over all cover up—except eyelids, if you already have a base on your eyelids. Pat the foundation under your chin, slightly, but not on your neck. Blend well at this point, even though your foundation is as close as possible to your natural skin tone. (To effect this, you might buy two shades, one a little darker than the other, and blend them yourself. For a guide as to shade, see chart on pages 104 and 105.

4. If you wear a cream rouge, apply it now under the cheekbones for a hollowed look. I like rouges in brown tones because they are more natural and don't impart that Baby Jane look. Again, *pat* on the rouge.

5. Including eyelids, powder your entire face, using translucent powder (never tinted). Use a cotton ball, which is cleaner than a powder puff and can be thrown away after use. Powder your face with downward strokes. You may have heard that all makeup should be applied in an upward motion, but downward strokes are used with powder because facial hairs grow downward. Like velvet, if rubbed the wrong way, the skin will not look smooth.

6. If you use a powder blush, apply this now, under your cheekbones in an upward motion—from middle of cheek to temple. Why "up" with blush and "down" with powder? Most of the peach fuzz grows low on the face, below the cheekbone. Ever notice that men don't shave on their cheekbones? The beard grows only in the jaw area.

7. If needed, fill in eyebrows with a pencil, using short, upward, hair-like strokes. Pencil color should not be much darker than hair color.

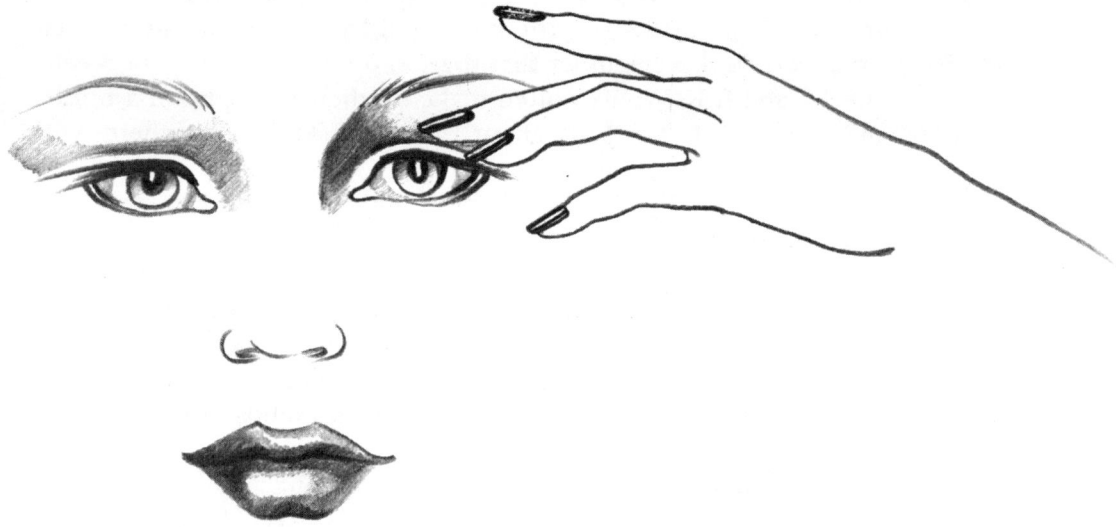

8. Heavy eyeliner, despite King Tut's current popularity, is now definitely passé. However, a smudged-on eyeliner can be used sparingly in brown or gray, and be sure to smudge away its hard line. I'm glad the hard eyeliner look is "out"—it tends to close the look of the eye and, I've always thought, cheapens a woman's appearance.

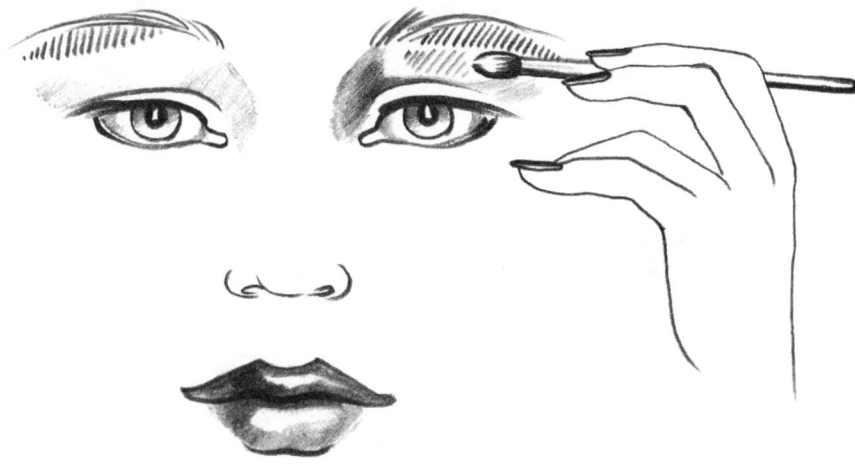

9. Eyeshadow should be applied in four places—each in a different shade. (1) Brush a light shadow under the brow. (2) Then, on the orbital bone, a dark pink or rose, and smudge in. (3) For the lid itself, use a pale shade or light earth brown, depending on your eye color. (4) Now brush in your smoky charcoal, gray, or dark brown, in between the orbital bone and eyelid (called the crease). Don't forget to smudge and blend. If you like, you can use a very little under the eye to balance the look.

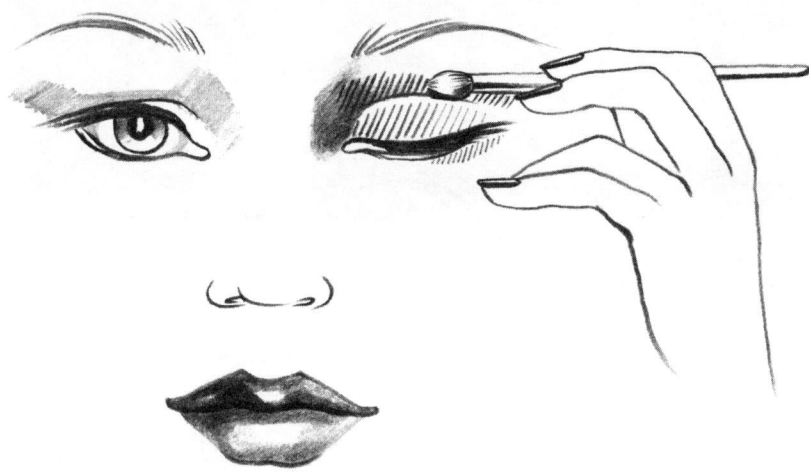

When shadowing your eyes, remember that light expands and dark contracts; therefore, shades lighter than your skin color will "bring out" an area, while a darker shade makes hollows. Light shadow (never white under dark eyebrows) is applied directly under the brow to give the illusion of a larger eye. If your eye is heavy lidded, a dark brown usually works well in the crease of the eyelid, as does gray. (Gray is especially good for blue eyes.) If you're unsure about color above the eye, stay with earthy tones—you can't go wrong with them.

10. Curl your lashes with an eyelash curler. Be sure to steady your arm on a fixed object to prevent involuntary movement.

11. Mascara in brown or black works best for everyone; colored mascaras are unnatural looking and hard to work with. Before you apply it, brush your lashes with powder; this thickens them. For even thicker lashes, apply both powder and mascara a second time. Do both the upper and lower lashes and work for a balance between both. To keep mascara on bottom lashes from dripping onto your face, dip a Q-Tip in powder and roll it upward under the lashes, drying the mascara. If a drop gets on the skin beneath your eye, dip a Q-Tip in your makeup base, then roll it over the mascara blob in an upward motion, curling lashes as you go. Always remove mascara before going to bed. Leaving it on overnight can cause your lashes to break, and sometimes creates an irritation.

12. Before applying lipstick, cover your lips with foundation, then brush lightly with powder. This will make lip color set better. Using a lip pencil, outline your lips with a slightly darker shade, which gives the mouth a nice definition. Fill in with color and gloss. Never use gloss as the outline, as it tends to run. You can make your own gloss by mixing food color with Vaseline—or mashing a little lipstick in Vaseline. When making up your lips, remember that there must be balance—the same prominence in your eyes and cheeks should be carried out in your mouth.

13. With a $1\frac{1}{2}''$ sable brush, go over the entire face in a downward motion, removing any excess powder.

Voila! You are now a siren!

COLOR CHART

Foundation Tones	Rouge Tones	Eyeshadow Colors
Blonde Ivory or light beige—should be the color tone of your skin. For contouring, mix 2 shades of darker color with regular foundation.	Light earthy tones, such as copper with a touch of pink.	LID: Pale shades of beige, taupe, or pale earthy tones. CREASE: Dark brown if lid is beige or taupe. Charcoal if lid is soft gray, blue, or green.
Brownette Same shade as your skin. If ruddy complexion, use beige with *no pink*. If sallow, use tone with a touch of peach color.	Earthy colors—coffee or rust or copper.	LID: Soft beige or taupe. CREASE: Dark brown. Next to Brow: Light beige, very light pink or light peach.
Brunette Most brunettes have a sallow complexion, so use a base with rose or peach. Stay with the tone of your skin.	Pink tones to color a sallow skin. Also peach.	LID: Soft lavendar or pale pink. CREASE: Charcoal or smoky tones.
Red Ivory or soft beige.	Earthy tones—coffee or copper.	LIDS: Earthy brown tones Perhaps a hint of avocado-green. CREASE: Stay with dark brown.
Black Skin Same color tone of skin, with peach added.	Copper tones, burgundy, or dark pinks.	LID: Light or dark brown, depending on skin color. Nothing too pale, which would make eyes look protruding. *Never white;* use peach, taupe, or light beige. Mocha on orbital bone. CREASE: Dark or light brown.

Lipstick and Gloss Tones	Daytime Look	Evening Look
Stay with the soft, natural shades. Line lips with a shade darker lipstick or lip pencil.	Stay soft and natural, with brown tones. Not too much color on eyes.	Deeper charcoal, or smoky, or dark brown shadow in the crease of eyelids and blend outward. The depth should be at outer corner.
If complexion is fair, stay with soft colors. If complexion is dark, lipstick or gloss can be darker.	Stay with brown tones, soft and natural.	Deepen eyelid crease with dark brown—depth should be at outer corner. If eyes are brown, stay with different shades of brown.
Depending on darkness of skin, use dark pink or light pink. No bright colors. Line lips with auburn eyebrow pencil. Stay with rusts, browns, coffee, copper.	Charcoal in the crease, and pale tones on the lid. Soft browns and dark browns.	Deeper charcoal in the crease—depth should be at out corner and a little under the eye. Slate with a little blue on lid. Don't forget to blend. Deepen crease, with depth at outer edge. Brush avocado-green under eye.
Depending on darkness of skin, stay with earth and rust colors. If lips are large, do not use gloss. Use a brownish lipstick with a touch of peach or pink.	Stay soft and subtle. Keep same intensity on eyes, lips, and cheeks.	Dark brown in the crease, a lot of depth in outer corner. Avocado on lid and under eye. Coppers and rusts also good on lids. As black skin is naturally toned and colored beautifully, a lot of makeup base is unnecessary.

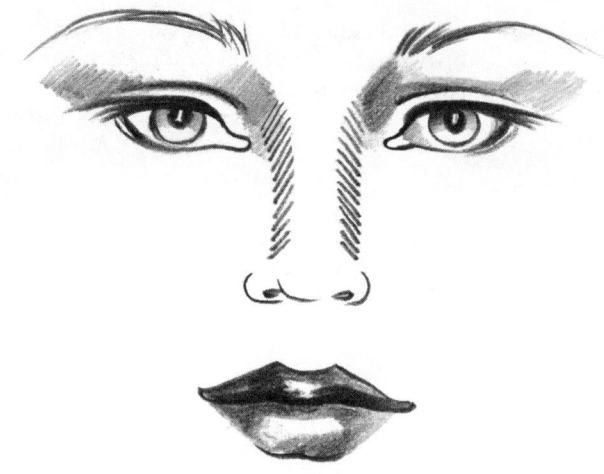

PROBLEM AREAS

Nose

If your nose is *too broad,* apply a slightly darker base in a thin line down each side of the nose, then blend foundation over it. This will give your nose a slimmer appearance.

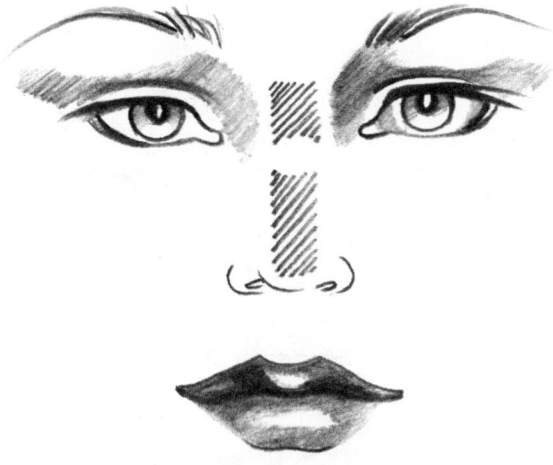

If your nose has a *bump,* you can make it look straighter by using a line of lighter foundation down the bridge of the nose in a straight line—but not on the bump. Remember to blend it.

If your nose is *too long,* touch a little dark makeup on the tip underneath—in the area between the nostrils—with an upward motion. Blend.

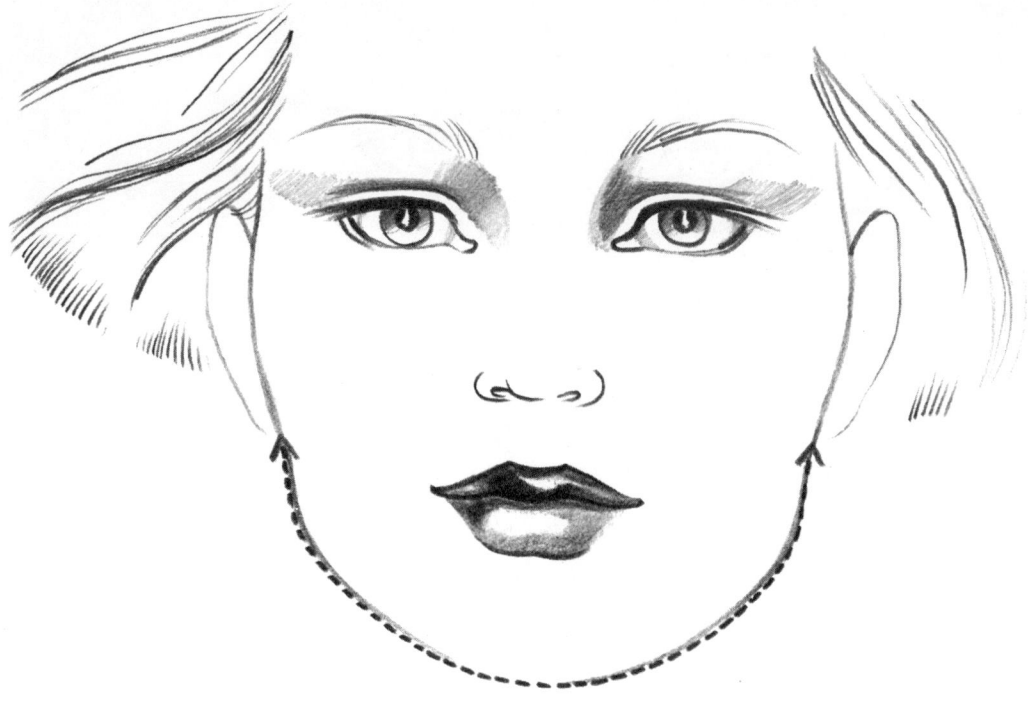

Chin

For a *weak chin,* use a lighter foundation all along the jawbone area. (Light expands and dark contracts.) Be sure to blend well with your fingertips so that there is no line of demarcation.

For a *prominent chin,* apply a darker foundation along the jaw area.

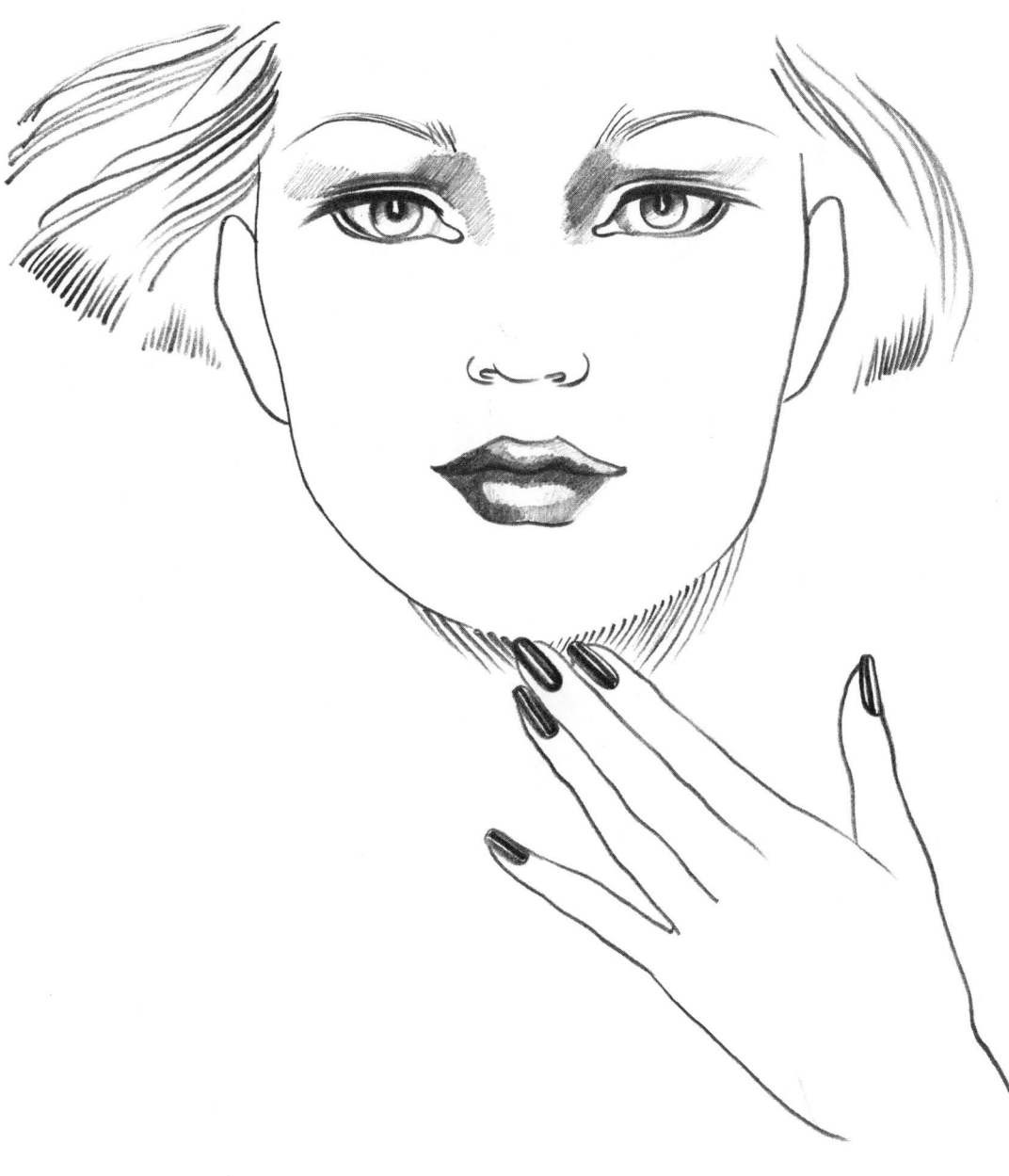

For a *wide jaw,* use a darker foundation from below the ear across the jaw line. Again, be sure to blend.

For a *double chin,* use a darker foundation under the chin, starting at the jaw line, and on jowl area, then blend. Afterward, blend your regular shade of foundation over this, and powder with a brush. Use a cotton ball or brush to remove excess powder.

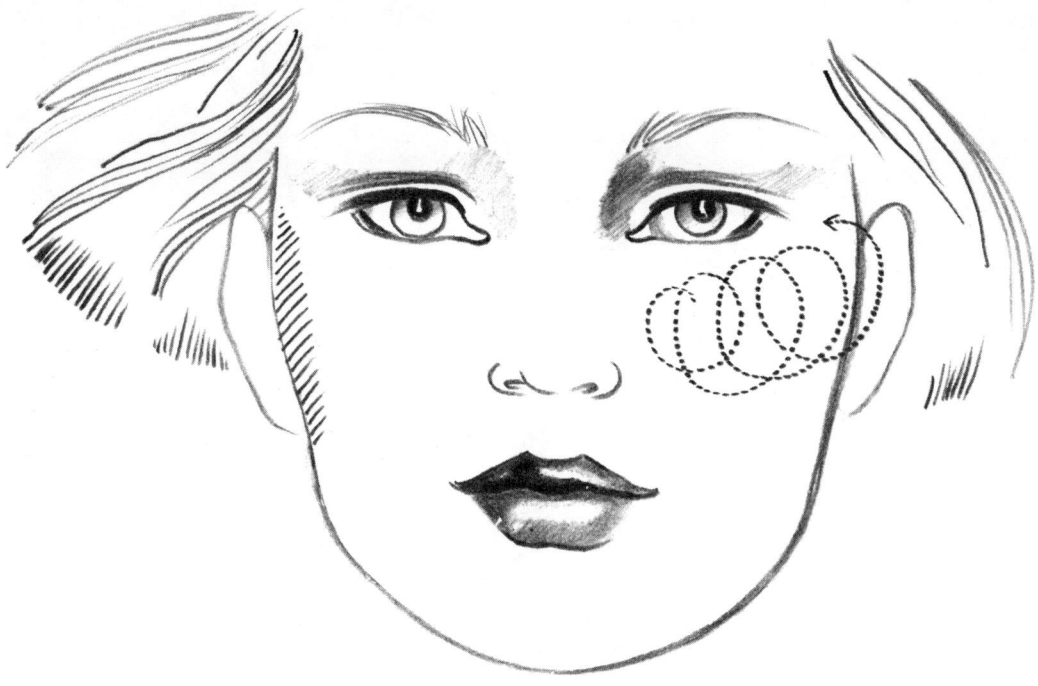

Narrow Face

Use a lighter makeup at sides of face, and bring rouge in circles out to the sides of your face, thus expanding it. Bring all eye makeup up and out from the eyes, giving an illusion of width.

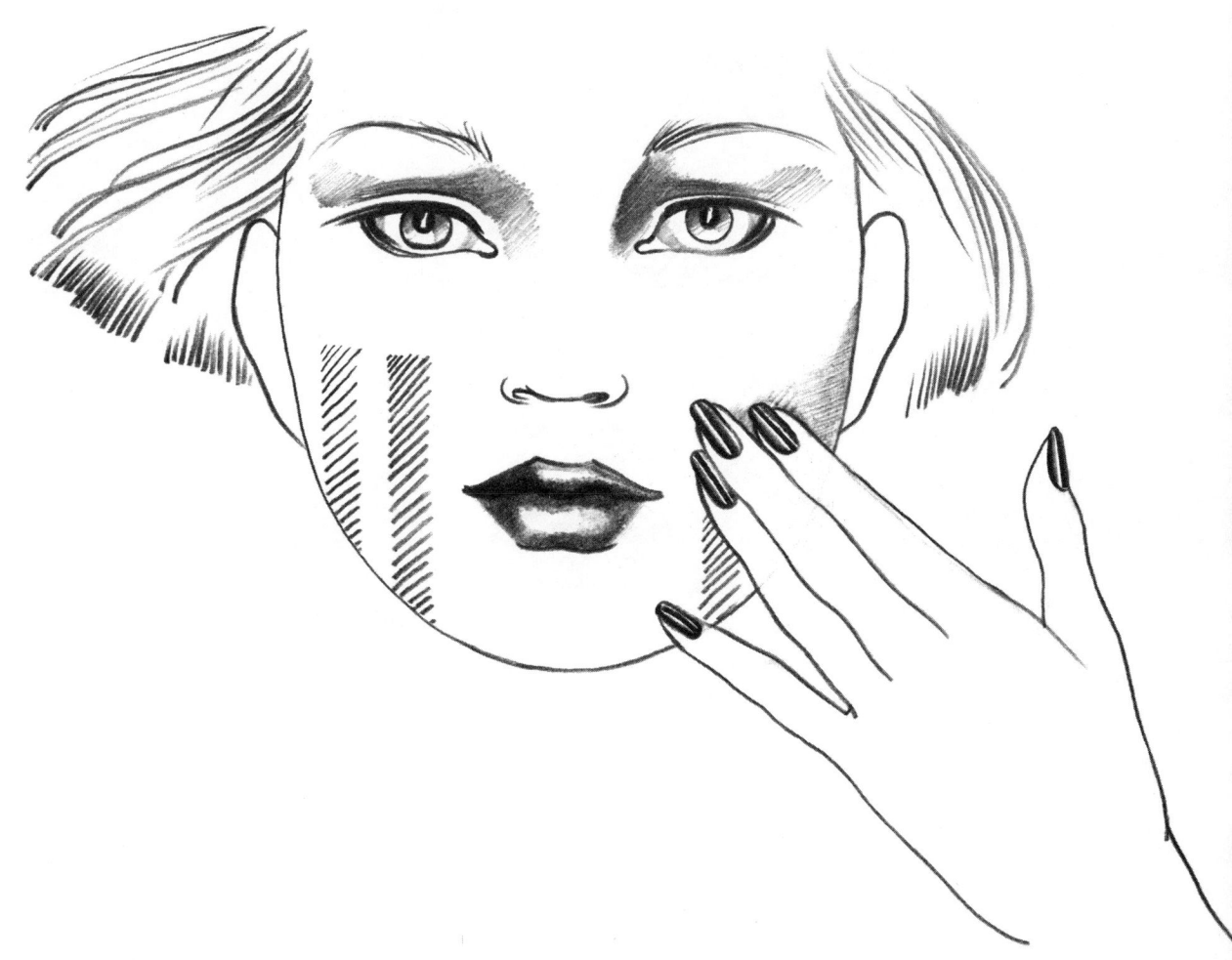

Round Face

With a darker makeup, draw two vertical, parallel lines from below the cheekbones out to the jaw bone, and blend this color down and out to your ear area.

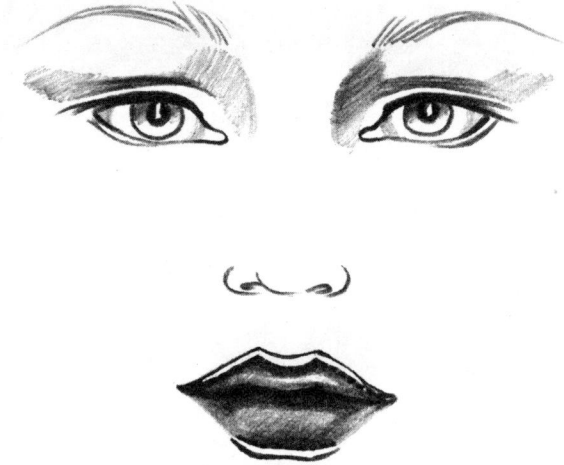

Lips

For *thin lips,* a darker shade of lipstick makes your lip line appear to recede, so use a rust, toast, or earth color. Outline the lips in one of these colors with your pencil, exceeding the natural line just a little. Then blend the line and lip color carefully so that your natural lip does not show through. Apply gloss only in the center of your mouth, thereby highlighting the fullest area.

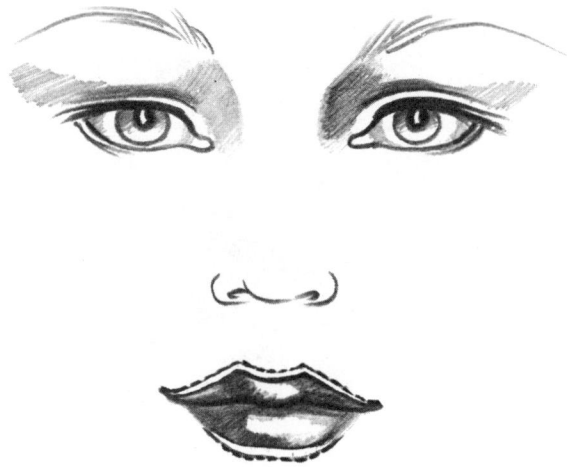

For *full lips,* line the lower lip just inside your natural lip, extending the line a fraction beyond the outer corners of the lips. By slightly elongating them, lips will appear less full. Do the same for the upper lip. Use a deep shade of lipstick, if deep colors look well with your skin tone. Do not use gloss, as this makes lips more prominent.

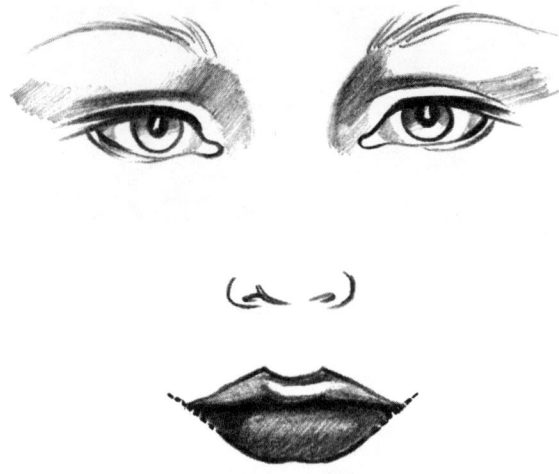

Most of us have *irregular lips,* one fuller than the other. This is easily remedied with the use of a lip pencil. Line the fuller lip just inside its natural contour; then line the thinner lip as it is. Use a deeper shade on the fuller lip; a lighter one on the narrow. These should be the same color tone so that the difference will not be noticeable.

If your *mouth droops* at the corners, extend the outline of the lower lip slightly upward, and outline your lower lip to focus attention there instead of at the corners. Use a darker shade on the lower lip, and gloss only in the center of the upper lip.

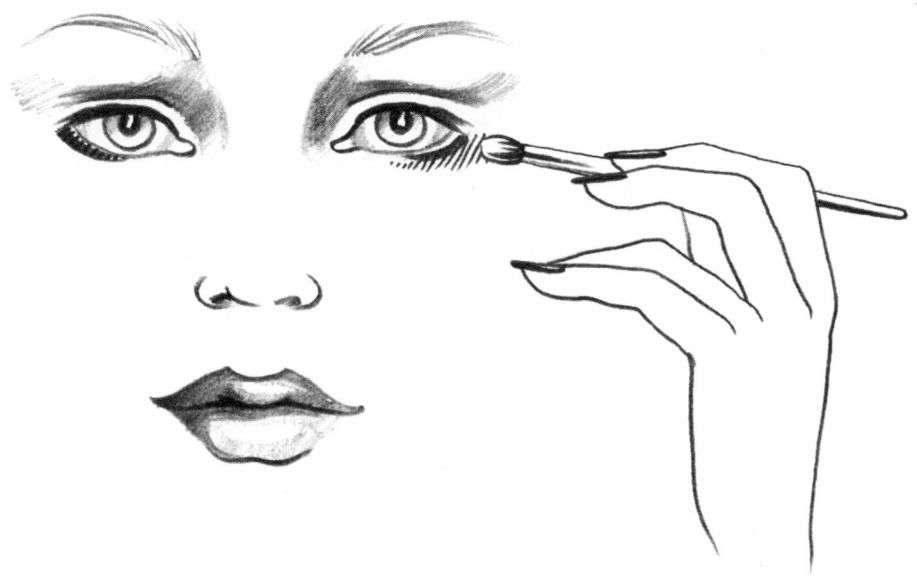

Eyes

Before beginning any eye makeup, apply a base from brow to lash, then powder slightly. This prepares the eyes for makeup, plus blending out any discoloration. It's like priming a canvas before painting a picture.

For *small eyes,* use a pale eyelid color to give the illusion of more eyelid space. Smudge a dark smoky color in the crease. Always blend with fingertips to avoid a line of demarcation. I like to use a mocha or a whisper of dark pink on the orbital bone to highlight the bone structure. Again, blending is imperative. Use smoky shadow under the eyes as well, brushing from the outer corner halfway toward the nose (*all* the way would tend to close the eye). Use a dark brow pencil to line at the base of the lash, making the lash appear fuller. Don't forget to smudge.

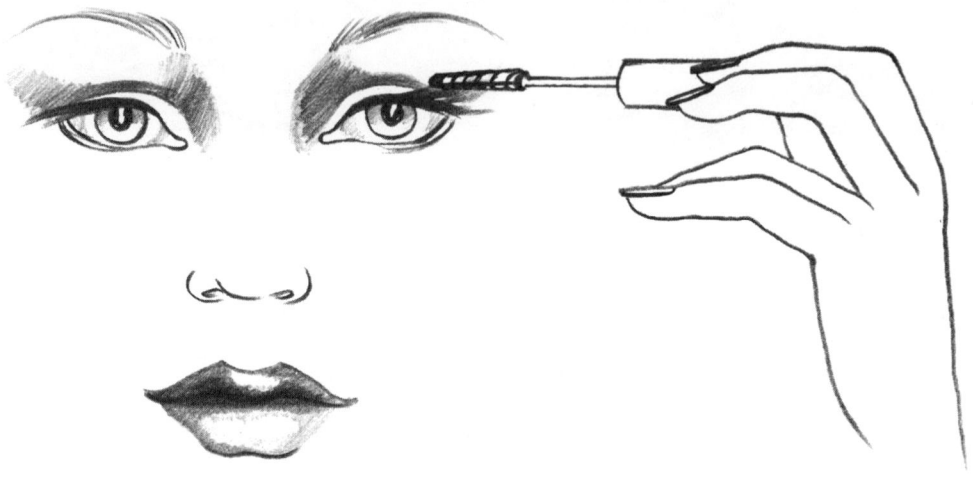

For *deepset eyes,* the eyelid color should be palest near the lash, both above and slightly under the eye. A smoky color of shadow is best, gray or charcoal for blondes and green for blue-eyed women—dark brown for brownettes, redheads, and brown-eyed women. Again use a dark brown soft pencil to line at the base of the lash, to make the lash appear fuller. Eyeliner *can* be used, but it mustn't look like a line—it should be applied and smudged with fingertips so that only a hint is apparent. Use a lot of mascara, and perhaps a demi lash.

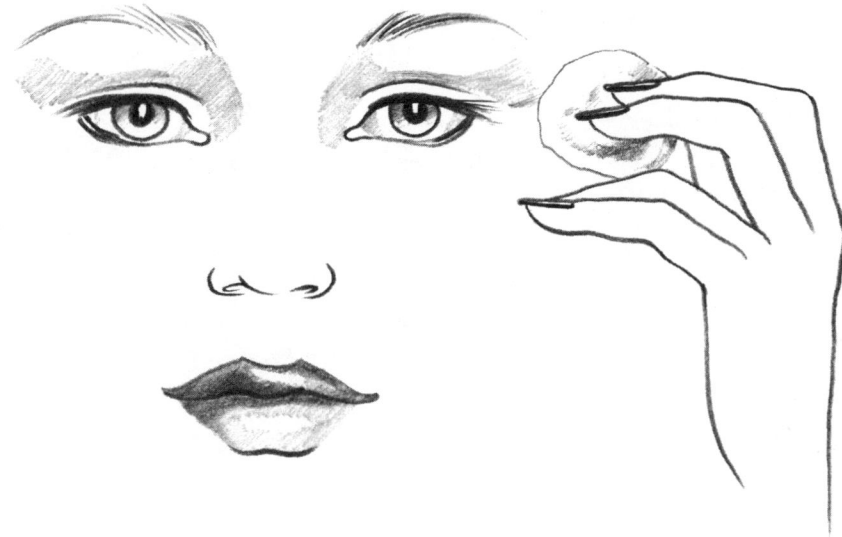

For *protruding eyes,* browns and smoky shadows are best, detracting from puffy or protruding eyes. Use subtle and muted shades, never a frosted shadow. Use a pale shade just next to the lash, but bring your smoky color or brown over the rest of the eyelid, making it appear to recede. A peach or soft beige can be used under the brow. Never use white; it is too obvious. Use a lot of mascara. Apply it, powder the lash lightly, then reapply mascara.

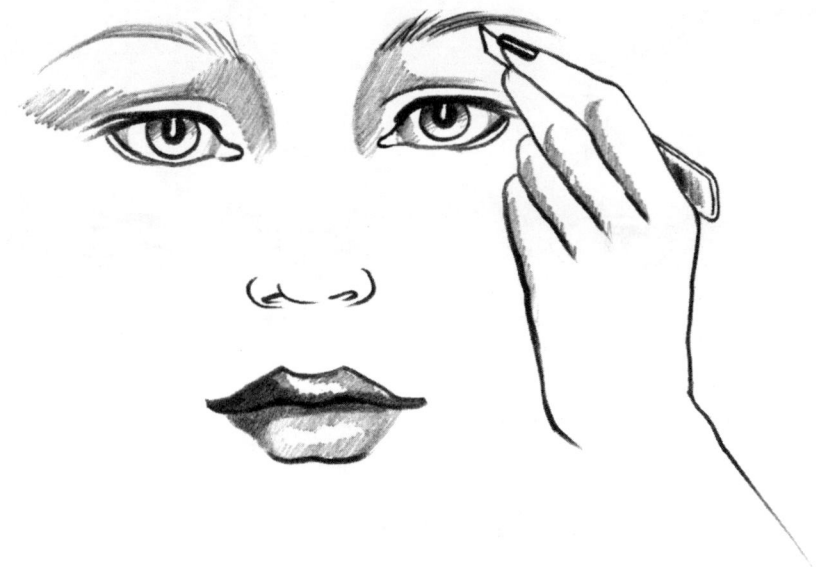

MORE ON EYEBROWS

Eyebrows shouldn't be too thin, too thick, too dark, or too light—any of which will detract from the eyes.

Locate your orbital bone by running a finger over your brow until you find the bony protrusion. If there are a lot of hairs below this ridge, you need to do some plucking—and I stress *some*. Do it only from underneath, and if necessary between the eyebrows or at the outer corners—never from above. Follow your natural brow shape. Unnatural lines and artificially arched eyebrows are unattractive. The brow should be about the same width from the beginning to the top of the arch, and then taper to the outer end.

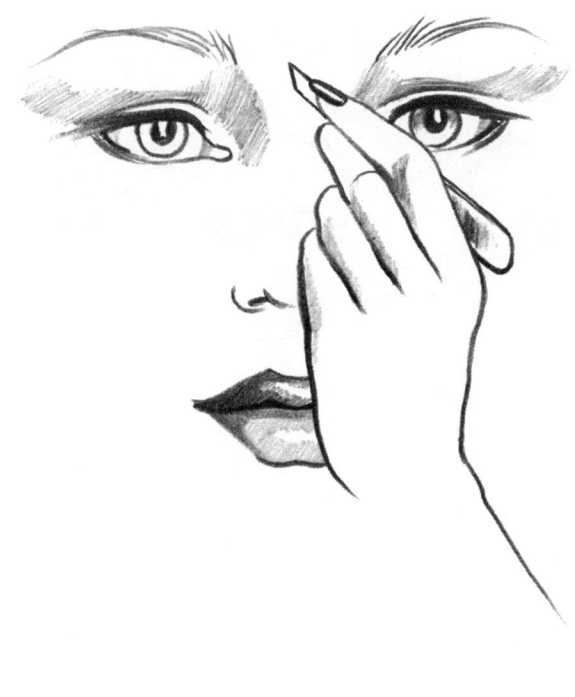

If your eyes are close together, pluck a few more hairs from the area between them, to give the illusion of a wider eyed look.

If your face is long, keep the brows straight, cutting the length of your face. A downward curve at the outer sides makes the face appear longer.

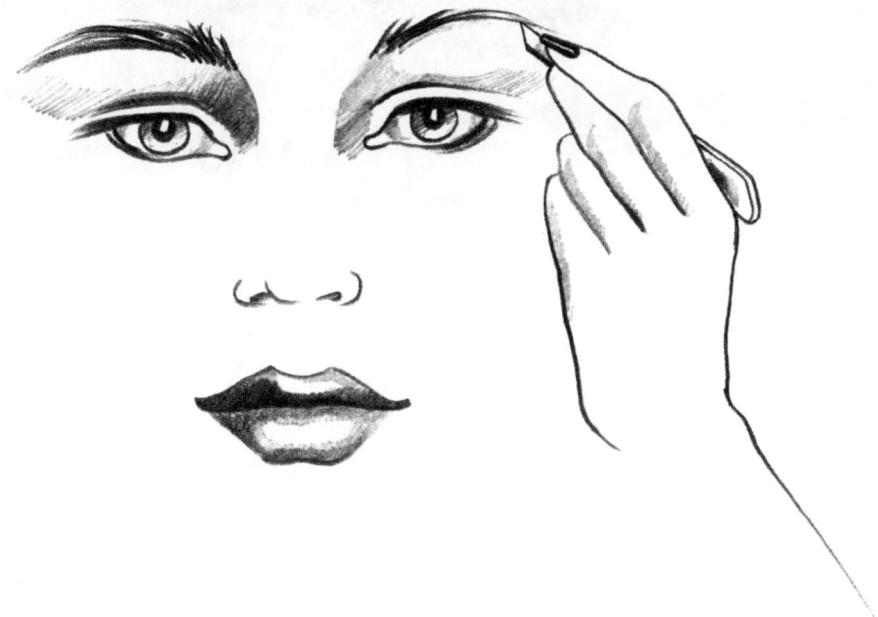

To make a round face longer, trim so that the arch is a bit more pronounced.

Too thick or bushy a brow closes the eye, making it look smaller. If you have this much eyebrow, get busy with tweezers.

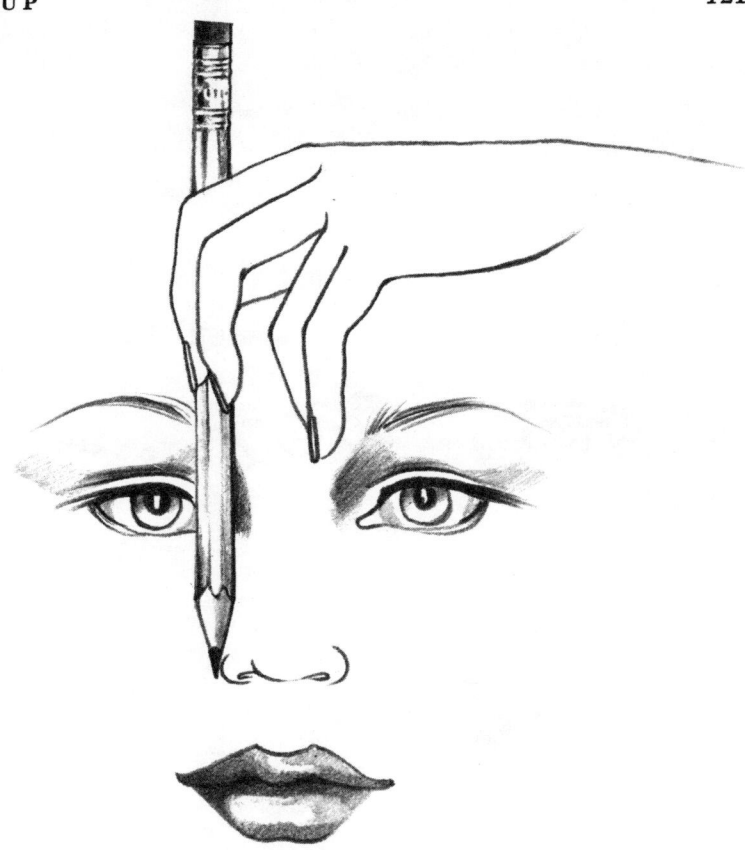

HOW TO TWEEZE

With a cotton ball, wipe the tweezers and the brow with alcohol, to sterilize. Brush the brows upward with a toothbrush, then back into place. Remove any hairs from between the eyebrows. Do not tweeze more from the center than necessary. For guidelines as to width, place a pencil with its tip at the side of your nostril and extend it straight up past the inside corner of the eye to the brow. Where the pencil touches at this point is the spot where eyebrow hairs should cease. Pluck only one hair at a time with a quick motion, in the same direction the hair grows. When finished, sterilize once more with alcohol.

If you can't manage the right shape on the first try, have it done professionally, after which you can do it yourself.

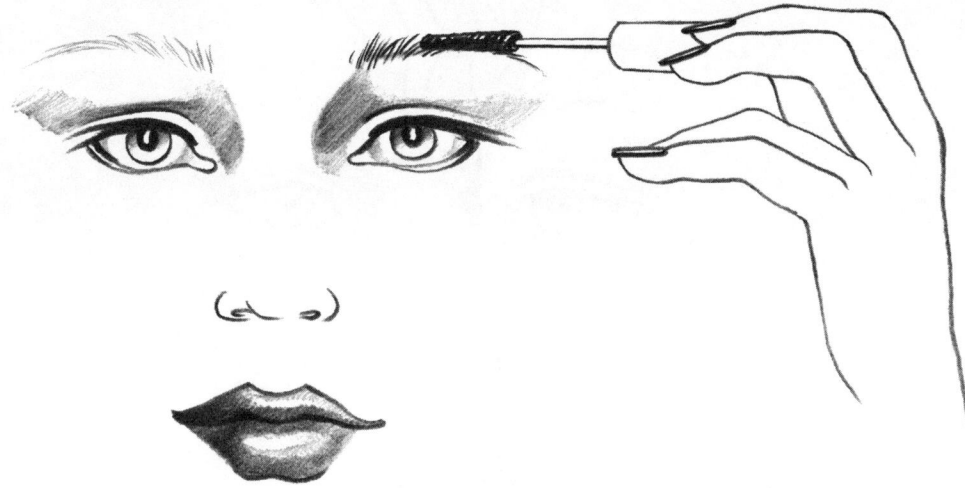

If your hair is dark, the brows should be a shade or two lighter. This can be done with an oil bleach or toner. If you have pale blond hair, the brows should be a touch darker; otherwise they'll be almost invisible. To darken pale eyebrows, use a light brown mascara. Remove most of the mascara from the brush before applying lightly—or have them dyed professionally.

PERSPIRATION

You have a problem if you perspire a lot on your face. The most common way women try to correct this is by covering their faces with powder, but too much powder makes them look like players in the Japanese Kabuki Theater.

The answer is simple. After you've applied translucent powder, dip a cotton ball in cold water, then pat (don't rub) it over your face. This removes excess powder and closes the pores so they won't continue emitting perspiration.

It may be a simple answer, but I went crazy trying to find it. In the heat of lights necessary on a sound stage, actors perspire freely and are forever having to be repowdered by makeup artists. The solution came to me when I was working on Mary Tyler Moore. With her great facial bone structure, Mary needs minimal makeup but, as with any actress, when she perspires the stage lights accentuate the shine. It was like a headlight the day I got my answer. Instead of the powder puff which tends to cake, I used loose powder and applied it with a brush, removing all excess powder afterward with the same brush.

We've already made powder puff two dirty words, but there *is* a use for it. There are three places on the face where we perspire more heavily—between the eyebrows, on each side of the nose, and on the chin. For these areas, use loose powder on a puff and press it in heavily. For the rest of the face, brush on your powder and remove the excess with a brush or a dampened cotton ball. The latter is good when you've been active and are overheated. Patting with a cotton ball, squeezed after dampened with ice water, is not only refreshing, it helps set your makeup.

So don't carry a compact. Carry loose powder stored in a small jar and a brush in your purse.

Joyce's own chapter has given you more complete information on the art of making up than anything I've ever read. You'll have to do a lot of experimenting, of course, but as she says, practice makes perfect. So have fun with your face, and be beautiful.

Now, to my department, the camera . . .

MAKEUP FOR PHOTOGRAPHY

Preparing for photography, stay natural and look like yourself. As with your hairdo for the camera, your makeup should stay natural. Powder yourself well in the "T area"—forehead, nose, and chin—because they grab the light. Make a matte finish on your face with powder. You can shade slightly heavier under the chin and in the hollows of your cheeks, because in black-and-white photography shading will show up as natural contours.

If your chin tends to doubling, you can minimize this for the camera by applying a foundation two shades darker than that used on your face, blending carefully along the jaw line. For still photos, Loretta Young used to use charcoal gray under her chin—almost black—and in the resultant pictures her face was full of light, the jaw line seeming to stand out from nothing. Very effective for photography, but not recommended for everyday.

If you're to be photographed in color, don't color so heavily that you'll look like a lady of the evening. Keep your skin tones natural and shade carefully. If you are lucky, your photographer will shoot a polaroid of you first, with which you can check your makeup. Take with you your loose powder and brush, as well as your foundation. The lights will likely make your face perspire and you'll need a retouch or two.

The angle at which you face the camera is very important. If you are heavy, or have broad shoulders, don't stand or sit straight on. Instead, turn your body so that you present a three-quarter angle to the camera, then turn your head to face it directly. If you have a double chin, you may think you should raise your chin to tighten the skin, but don't overdo it. When you raise your head too much, the camera looks up your nostrils. Instead, have the camera at eye level, or higher, thereby hiding the skin area beneath your chin, and keep your head straight on into the camera. If your face is round like mine, turn your head slightly to either side and look back at the lens. If chipmunk cheeks are a defect, you can always pose with your elbows on a table, then tuck your fists at the sides of your cheeks—a neat camouflage and a cute pose.

If the lights bother you to the extent you find yourself squinting or frowning, ask the photographer to co-operate with you. Close your eyes for a moment and allow your face to relax totally. Have the cameraman count to four before he snaps. If you open your eyes on his count of "three," you'll have a natural look when he clicks the shutter on "four."

One last hint. Keep your clothes as natural as your makeup. Wear something classic rather than outrageous so the photograph will stand the test of time. White is good around the face—a blouse or scarf. If your face is round, wear a V neckline. If long and narrow, wear a square or boat neckline. If your neck is short, don't scrunch it up in a turtleneck or cowl—give it a chance to show and look longer with a V neckline.

7
What's Your Top Figure?

Women with naturally good figures are just plain lucky. Everything hangs well on a good skeleton, and you can't make yourself a new one of those. A female with bones not too big nor too small, with wide shoulders, a tapering waist, and long, slim legs—she's got it made. She could wear a U. S. mail sack and look good.

I should be so lucky—I'm not—and so should you. If you're in my club, you'll have to work at making your figure the very best possible, on top of the bone structure God gave you.

Every bit of business that pads your bones can be changed and/or controlled in five ways. These are (1) your intake of food and liquid, (2) corrective exercises, (3) posture, (4) the clothes you wear, and (5) if you so choose, plastic surgery.

Here's the good news . . . I'm *not* going to give you a diet. You're already on one—which isn't really a diet, it's a matter of eating habits. You can eat your head off if you want to, as long as you opt for the correct foods.

I'll give you a far-out example. In the neighborhood of Tibet live a people called the Hunzas. Study of their diet reveals that they eat only fruits, vegetables, grains, seeds, and nuts—and drink a type of milk that's like yoghurt. (Twice a year during festivals, they slip up and have a yak steak.) Each spring, they go on a fast. Their longevity is among the longest on record; the women bear children well into middle age, sometimes sired by old boys in their 90s. And the Hunzas don't know the meaning of overweight. Got it?

Closer to home, my husband and I are another example. On our honeymoon in Montreal, the weather was so cold that we got little outdoor exercise. That fact, combined with fabulous French restaurants, added five pounds to my frame. I came home with the flu, spent a week in bed and added another two pounds. Seven pounds on 5' 11½" made me look as though I were inflated. In the following week, I ate according to Joyce's recommendations—and lost all seven pounds. That's when I leaned into Bill about his bad eating habits. He hadn't a weight problem but wasn't properly nourished. He used to go without eating all day, then would bring pizzas home. Or at 10 P.M. he'd say, "Let's eat a couple of cupcakes." Now we no longer have any junk food in the house. He eats a salad at lunch, and a well-balanced dinner, usually without dessert. He's forty years old now, looks thirty, and feels a lot better.

Diets, per se, are sort of dumb because the day you finish with any of them, you begin immediately to regain the weight you just worked so hard to lose. Keeping it off is harder than losing it. Diets are not only ineffectual because of this; they're actually bad for you. This is what happens. Oxygen is carried to the heart through coronary arteries, which are normally open and clear tubes. With frequent gain and loss of weight (and I'm talking about a simple ten pounds you might keep adding, then shedding), cholesterol deposits build up on the inner walls of the arteries, inviting heart attack. Every time you gain weight, these deposits are added and are *not* removed when you lose those pounds. Repeated weight gain and loss also results in the formation of fat deposits *on* the heart wall. Repeated diets make for a deadly process. How much safer and simpler it is to stay on a lifetime program of proper nutrition!

I'll give you a diet *not* to go on, ever . . . the liquid protein. The word protein comes from the Greek, and means primary. If it's of first importance, then how come all the scare about liquid protein? This diet has made a lot of people ill; has even caused death. It is not a natural diet. Those who've suffered through it have supplemented it with only water and/or coffee for several weeks. When on a liquid-protein diet, you lose potassium, and a dearth of potassium can make you faint, cause constipation, and have an irregular heart beat. People buying liquid protein have seldom been told they should take potassium every day, as well as folic acid, B complex, and vitamin C. Without these supplements, the system goes into shock. If you attempt a liquid-protein diet—or any diet, for that matter—without the constant vigil of your physician, you're being foolish.

Before I quit the subject of protein, there's something you should know about it that Joyce told me. The more protein you eat, the more calcium you need, because calcium and magnesium together help stabilize protein. Taken alone, protein leaves a toxic ash. Get your calcium and magnesium from vegetables. Any type of high-protein diet is dangerous. Example: Dr. Denis Burkitt, a renowned researcher, studied a group of African natives over a period of fifteen years. These people had a diet high in natural carbohydrates, vegetables, fruits, grains, and very little animal protein. They were healthy and had no incidence of cancer. When Dr. Burkitt put them on the American diet of high animal protein, refined foods, and sweets, they developed varicose veins, followed by hemorrhoids and diverticulosis, and ultimately, cancer of the colon. When he returned them to their natural diet, the symptoms and diseases were eliminated.

That's all I have to say about what you eat. Everything in this book regarding your intake, with the help of the charts in the Appendix, will steer you into eating habits that knock off—forever—the necessity of your ever again going on a diet to lose weight.

If you've stuck with it so far, your figure should be in top possible shape. If you haven't yet reached that high point, let me give you a tip about weighing yourself. Forget the daily scale check. When you're trying to lose weight, it's emotionally destructive to hit the scale every day and fret about it. If you've gained even a couple of ounces and are a compulsive eater, you may get upset and look for comfort in the wrong foods. Weigh yourself once a week only. Your true weight is in the morning, after you've eliminated and before you've eaten or drunk anything. Even a cup of tea or a glass of juice will show up five minutes later as one pound. Weight first thing in the morning is not only your true weight, it's your lightest, and discovering it will make you feel better. In the interim, you can tell how you're progressing by the way you feel and by the fit of your clothes. Professional models do weigh themselves every day, but if they learn they have gained even a few ounces over their minimal weight, they fast for one or two days to remove the excess weight before it becomes permanent. Unless you'd like to follow their example, don't make the scale a daily depressant.

EXERCISE

Exercise is necessary for your health, but not necessarily your weight. Exercise is not the catalyst it's cracked up to be. It won't banish many pounds, it will only redistribute weight. But it is important in that it will give you a firm body and good muscle tone. Fat is what you get when you sit around the house all day doing nothing.

You don't have to wear leotards or spend money at a gym. The cheapest and best exercise is walking. It's good for your heart, hips, calves, and thighs, it makes you feel great and helps clear your mind of emotional problems. I often walk with the dog for a half hour after dinner. If I'm lucky, my husband joins us for a threesome.

Jogging is free, too, but if you do it outdoors, don't jog on a hard surface—find a grassy stretch. Don't try for a mile the first day; rather, work up to a good distance gradually. Joyce jogs two to three miles every day to keep in shape. There is no better exercise than jogging. Not only will it help to maintain your weight, but it will rearrange your body as it should be and remove the lumps and bumps. Be sure you wear the right kind of shoes so you don't shock your vertebrae. Ask for jogging or running shoes. They are different from regular shoes.

My third suggestion is also free, except for the cost of a jump rope, which is easily packed and can go anywhere with you. Jumping rope is marvelous for circulation and all parts of the body. Work up to five minutes a day.

The fourth is a bit more expensive but very beneficial—a bicycle.

Before starting *any* exercise program, check with your doctor, most particularly if you've been slothing throughout most of your life.

CORRECTIVE EXERCISES

The daily exercises given you in Chapter 2 are for fitness and muscle tone. I do them at home or at my gym workout—after work, because my work makes me tense, and evening exercise relaxes me for a good night's sleep. Choose the time that's best for you.

Now for exercises to change your body. To decide what needs correction, stand before a mirror in the nude. I know, it takes courage to face yourself that way, but *do* it. Make a note of the areas that need trimming.

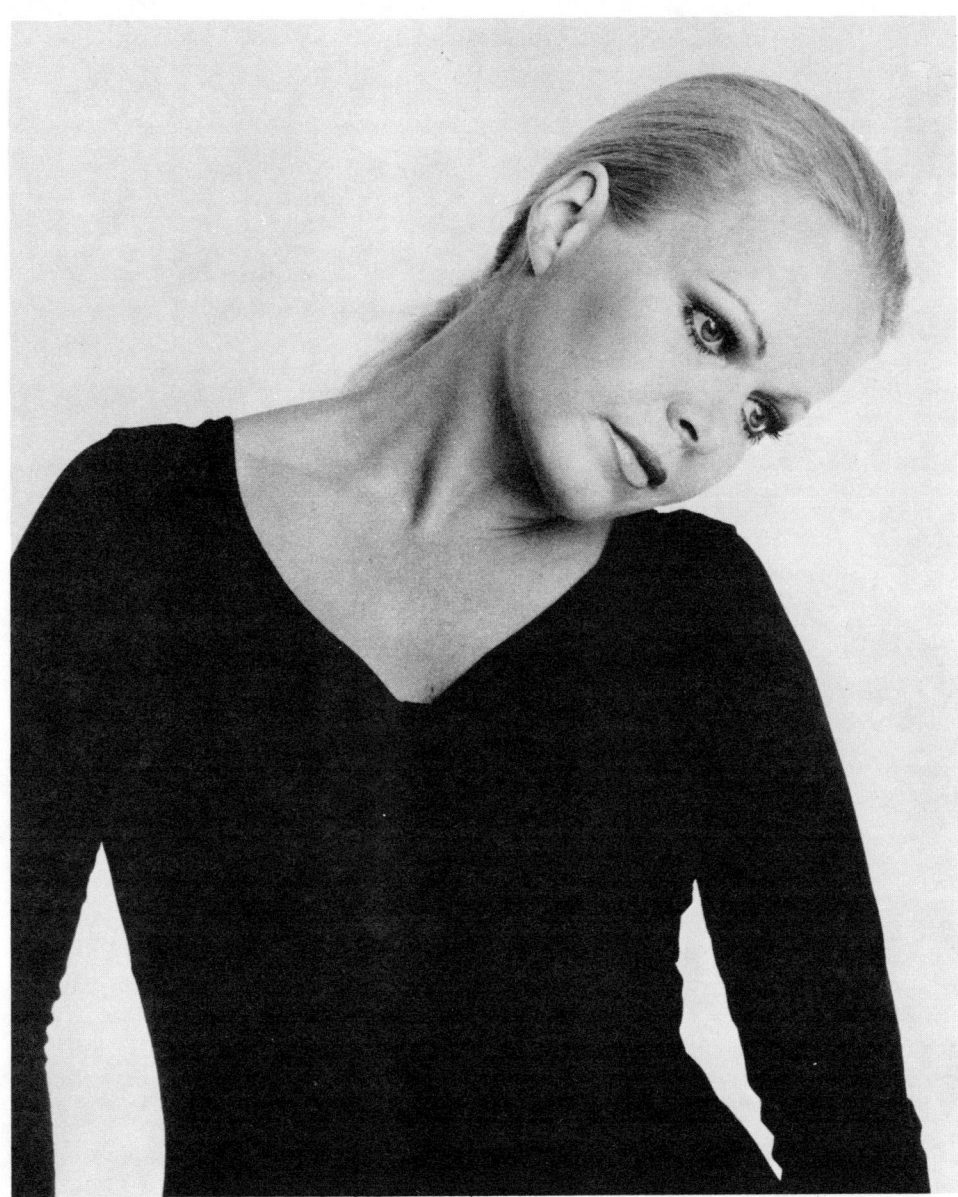

Neck

1. Keeping your shoulders down, stretch your neck by trying to touch ear to shoulder. Impossible, perhaps, but the attempt is great for neck muscles. Do 5 times on each side.

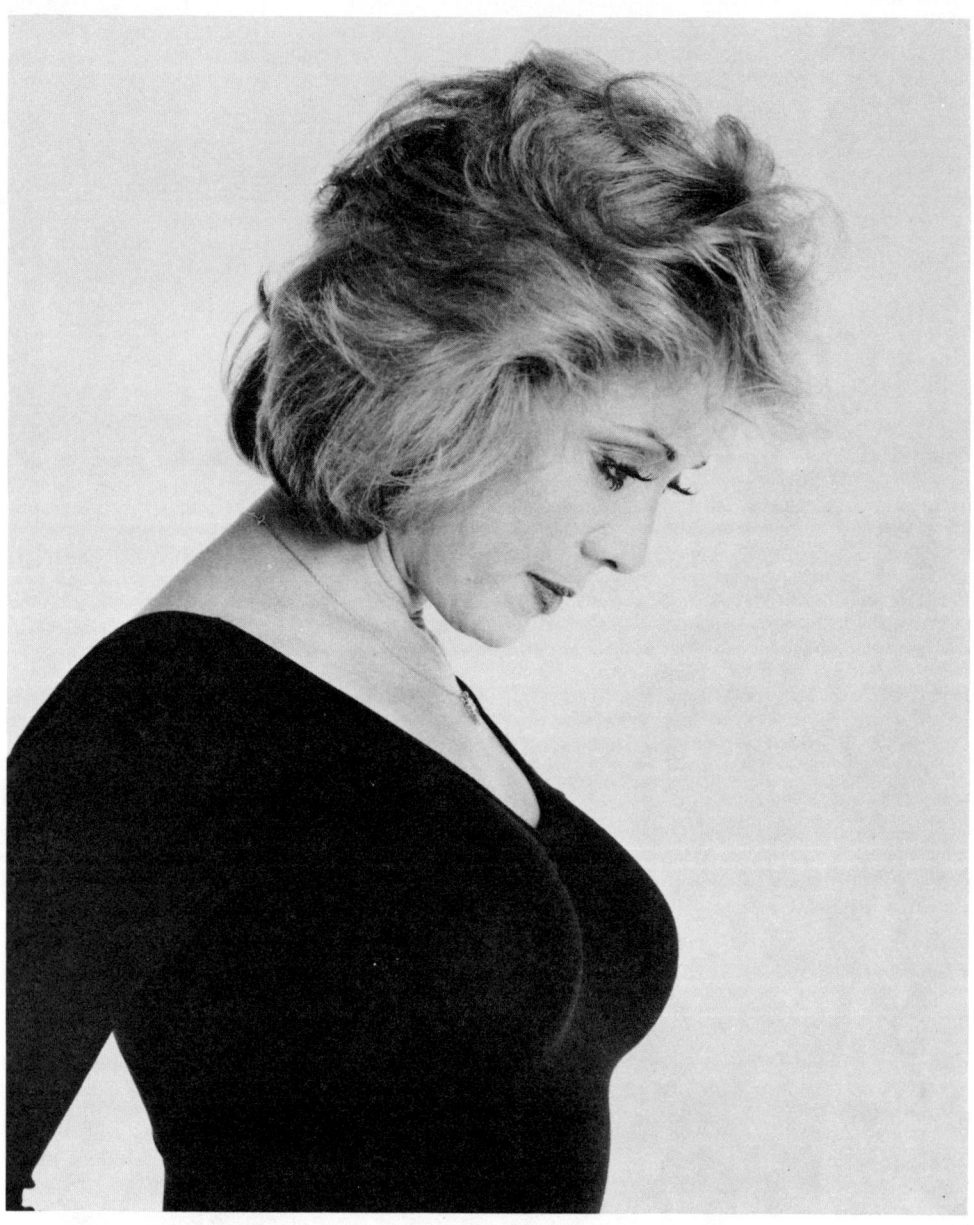

2. Drop your chin halfway to your chest, then roll your head from right to left, back and forth, 5 times. Do this *slowly*. Any quick motion

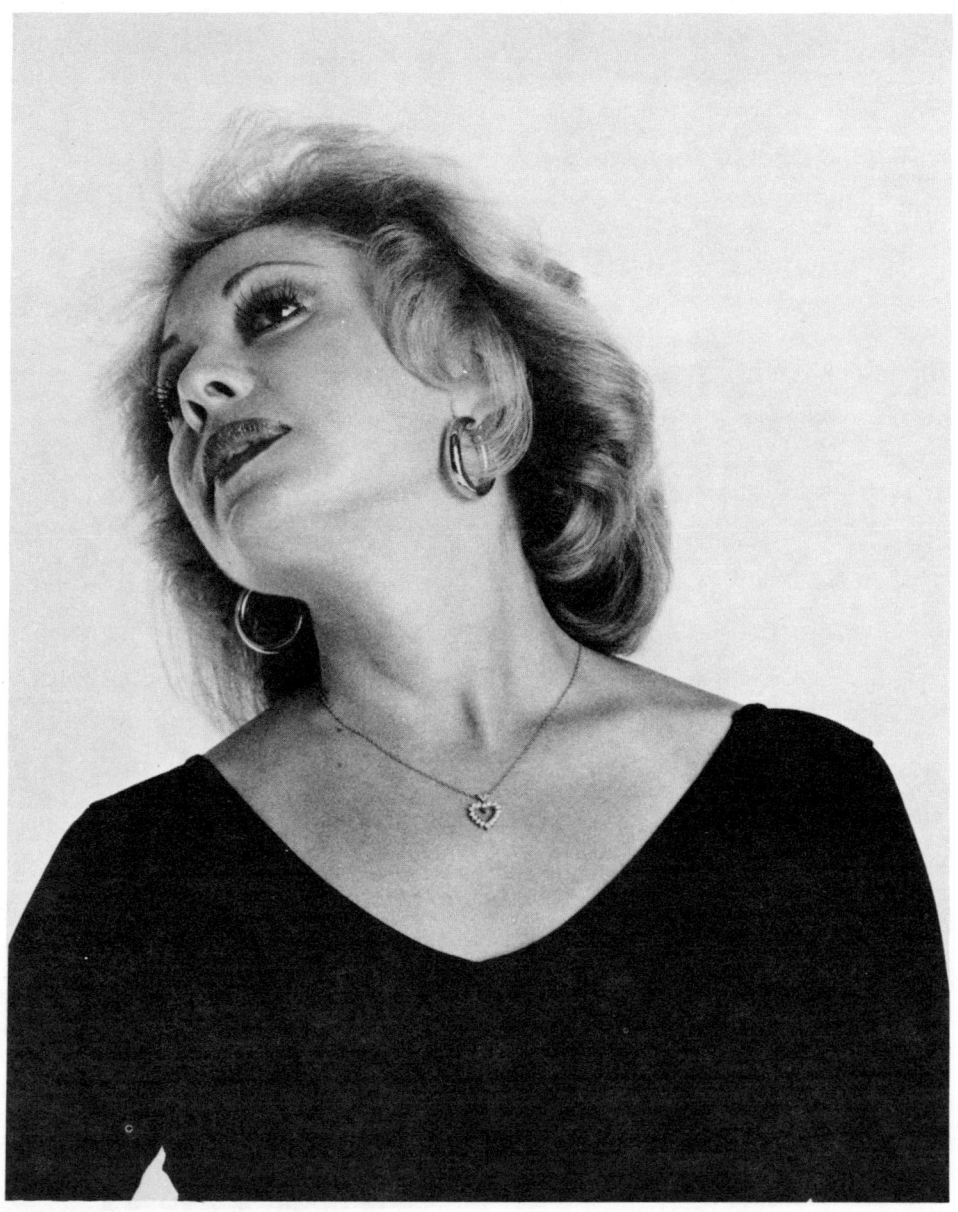

involving the neck puts a strain on the cervical spine and is asking for trouble.

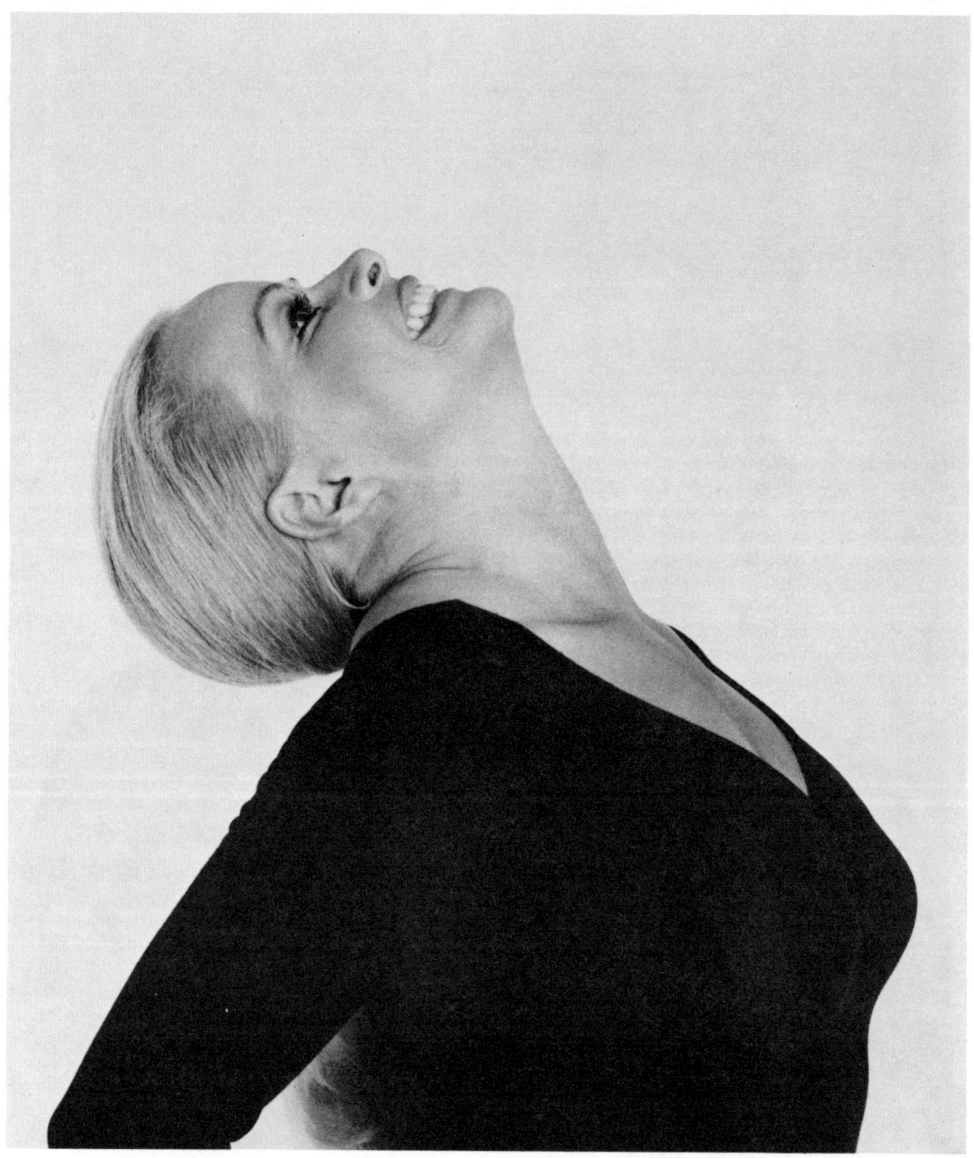

3. To make the neck supple and keep it from sagging, tilt your head back, then tighten muscles by grinning ferociously. Contract and relax 5 times. (Don't ever crack your neck for relief. I've gotten into this habit and must get out of it, because rubbing vertebrae against each other can build up calcium deposits and incur future neck problems.)

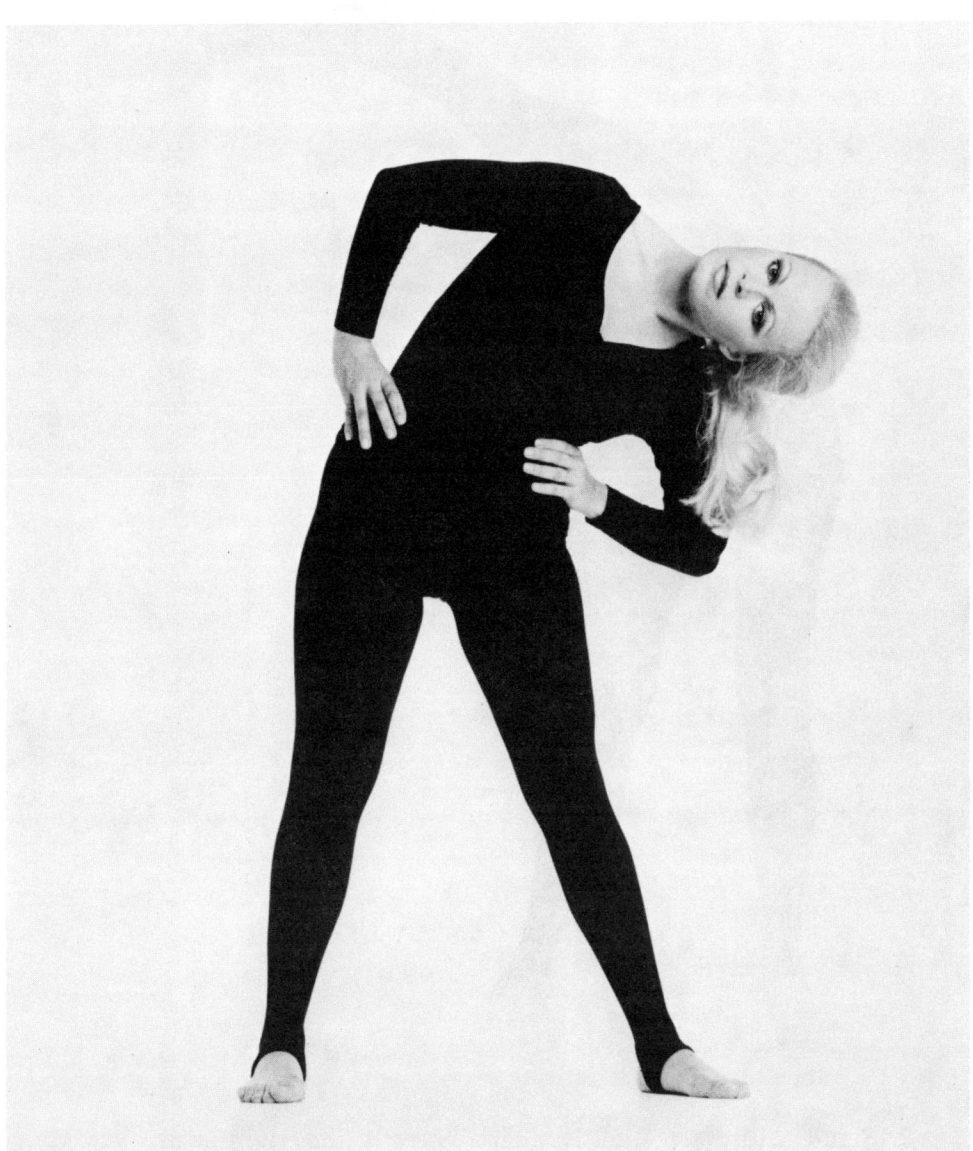

Waist and Torso

1. Stand erect with legs slightly apart and place hands on your waist. Circle the torso 10 times to the right, 10 to the left. While you rotate, concentrate on holding in your stomach and tighten those muscles. This exercise is a great waist slimmer and tummy tightener.

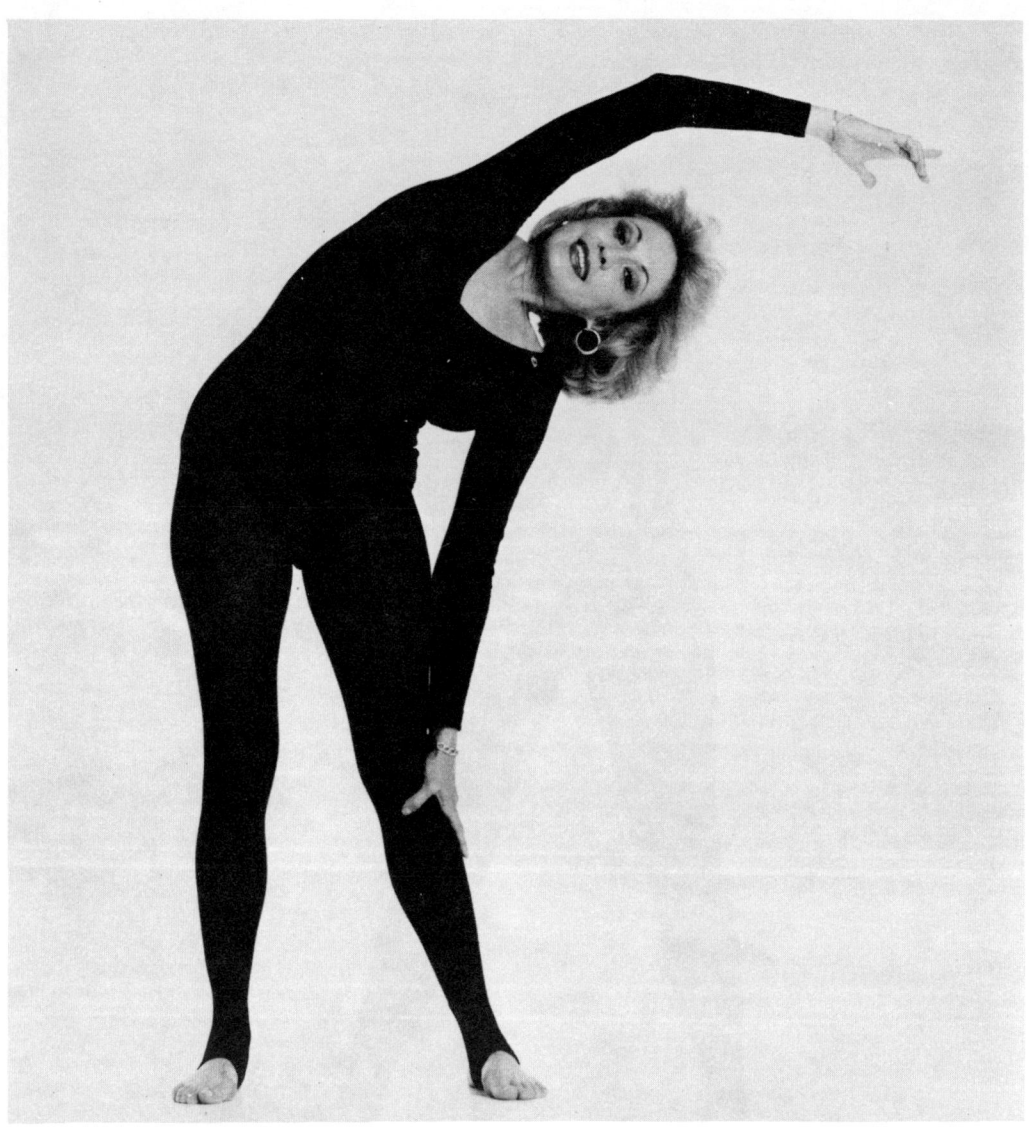

2. Stand with feet slightly apart. Stretch the right arm over your head and make an arc with your body by leaning far to the left. Do this 5 times on each side and work up to 10 each. This one pulls and tones the side area all the way from your hips to the underarm area.

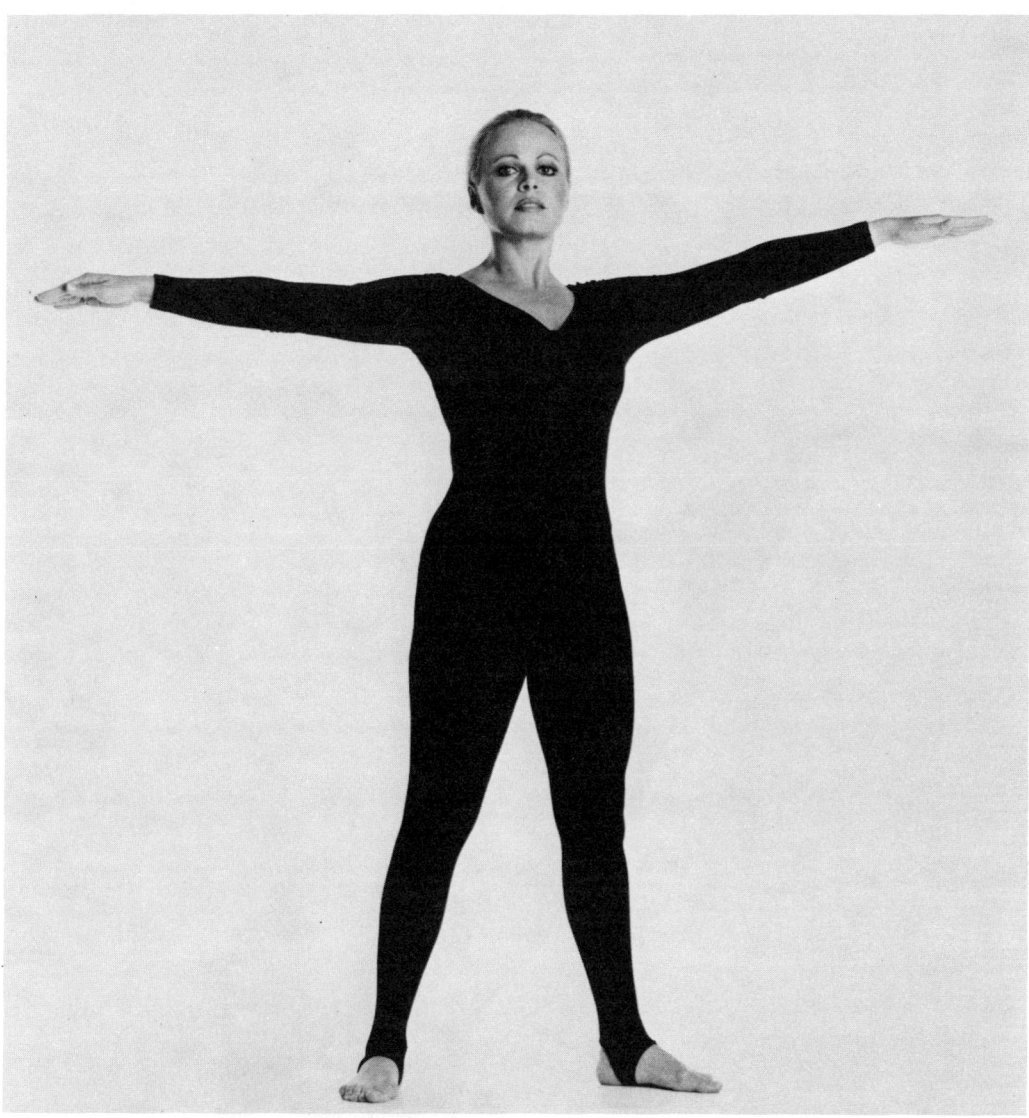

Arms

Arms are often neglected and prone to develop in later life into what my aunt calls "wattles."

1. With feet slightly apart, stretch arms sideways to shoulder level. Rotate them (simultaneously) forward 5 times, then backward for 5, making tiny, quick circles. Repeat, making larger circles. Gradually increase to 10 times each. This will help tighten any flab on the upper arms.

(If you have quite a bit of flab on the upper arms and can't tighten it with exercise, this *can* be corrected by plastic surgery. But know that it will leave a slight scar.)

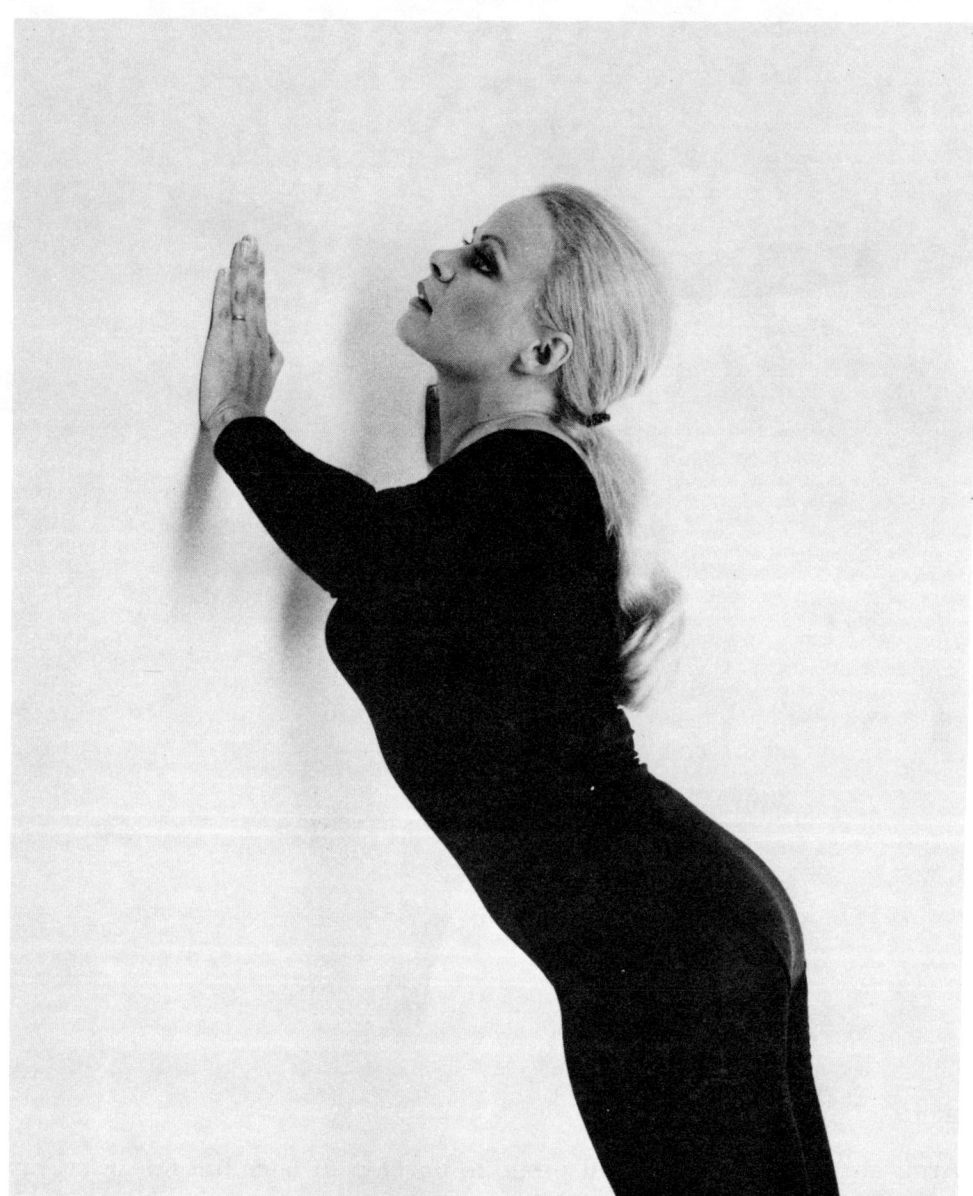

Bust

1. The best exercise for the bust is akin to doing pushups against a wall. Stand three feet away from a wall, place both hands on the wall, then

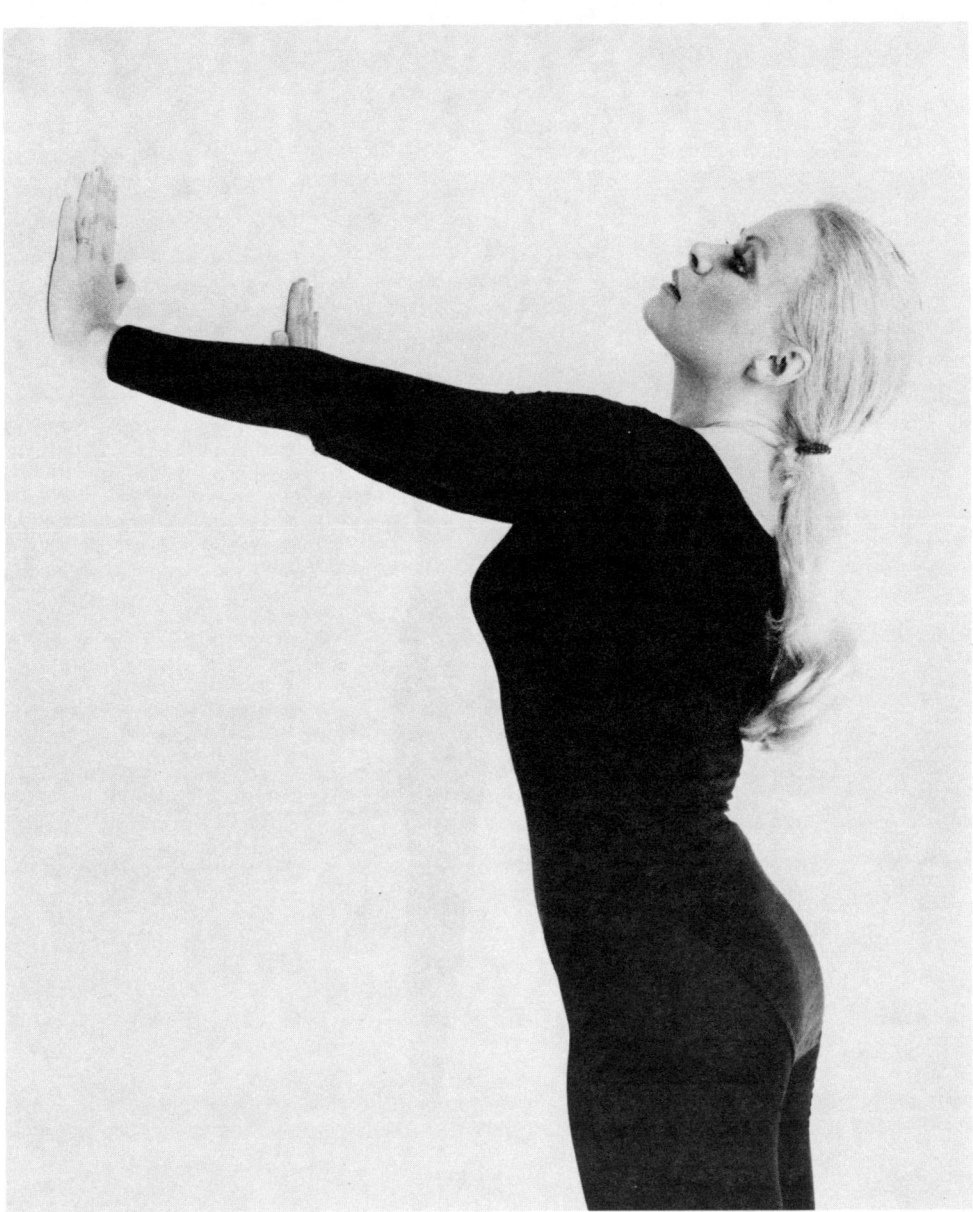

push yourself to and away from the wall. Doing this slowly enlarges, doing it fast decreases the bust.

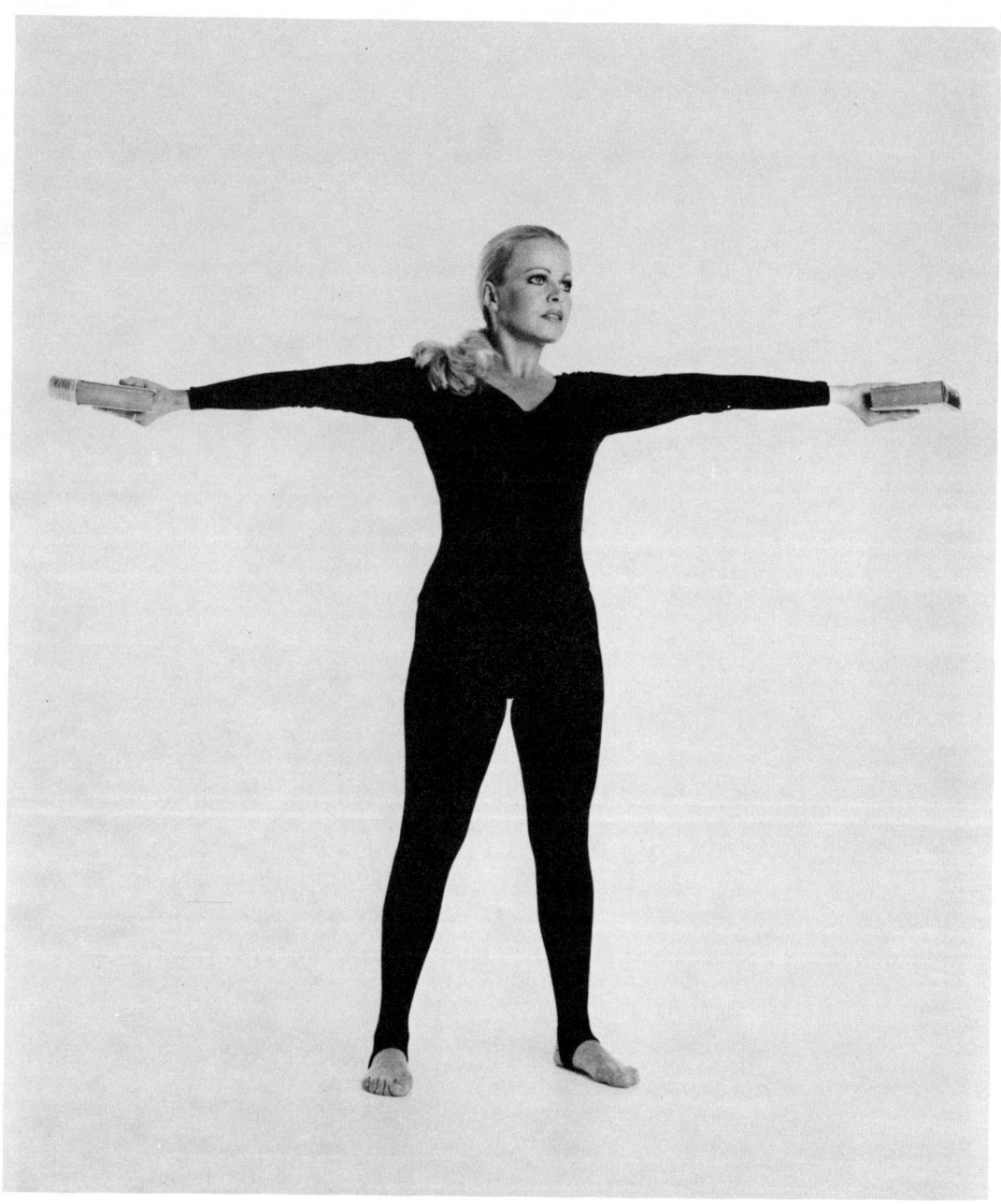

2. Hold a book in each hand. Slowly raise and lower arms, first at your sides, then in front of you. This strengthens pectoral and arm muscles,

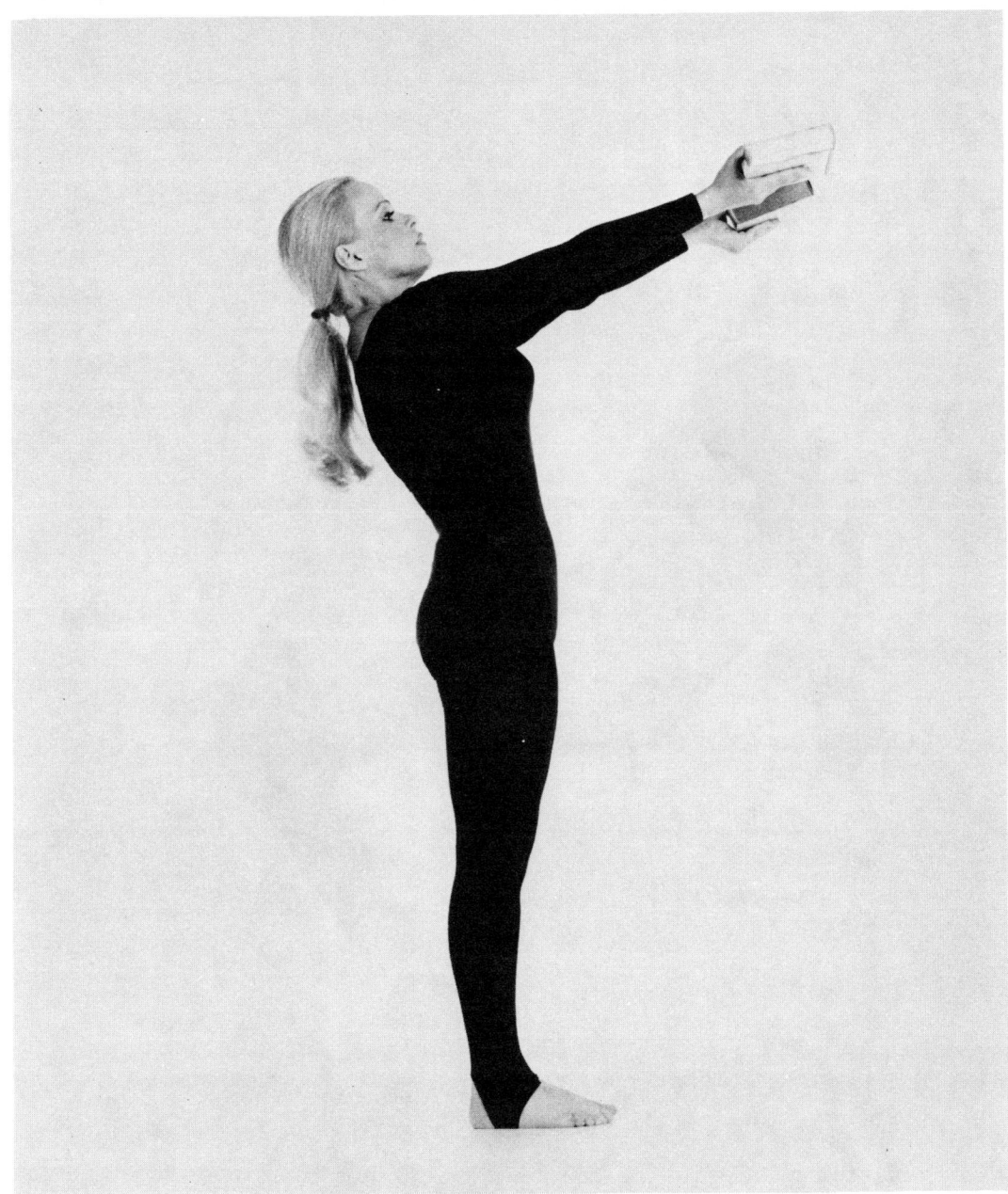

and is great for tennis buffs. (If your bust is quite small or overlarge, or there's a loss of muscle tone because of childbirth, you can think about plastic surgery, which will be discussed at the end of this chapter.)

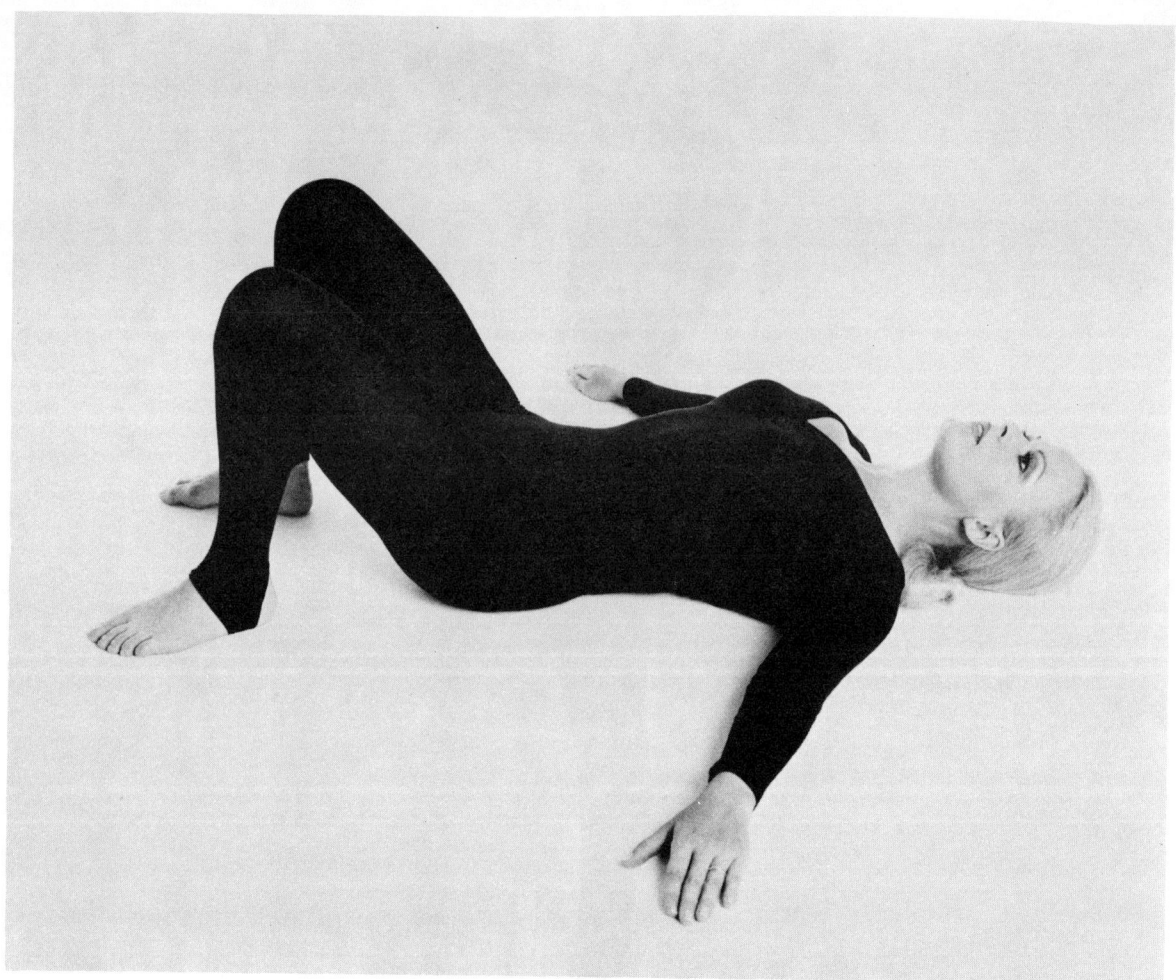

Hips

1. Lying on your back with arms out to the side, palms down, bring

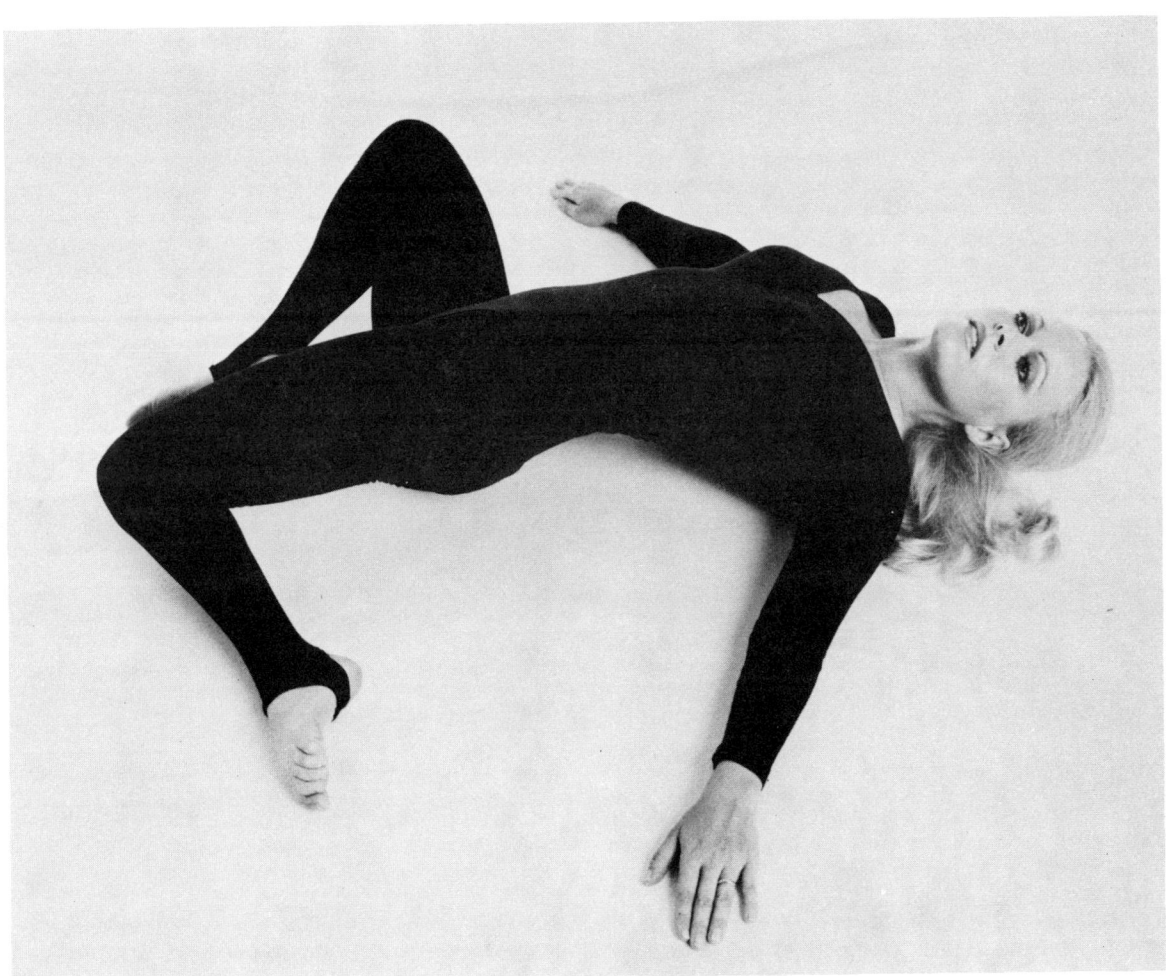

heels up to your buttocks, then twist both legs to the left, then right. Keep your back on the floor and move only the hips. Each side, 15 times.

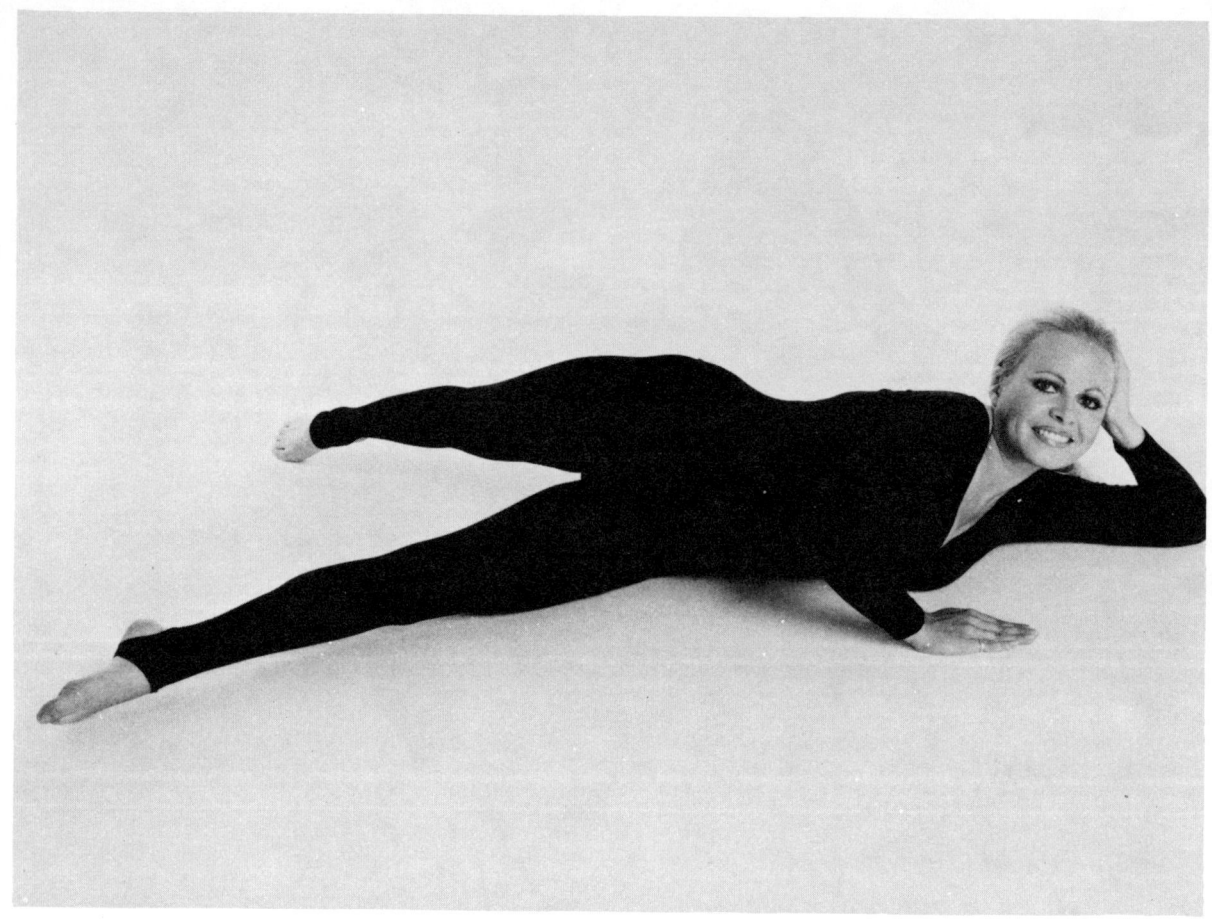

2. For bulges on hips or outer thigh. Lie on your left side with your head cushioned on your outstretched left arm and your right arm in front of you, palm on the floor for support. Scissor the legs 20 times. Repeat on your right side. Jogging is also good for the hips as it helps to tighten and pull the buttocks up.

Thighs

1. For bulges high on the outer thighs, do exercise No. 2 above.

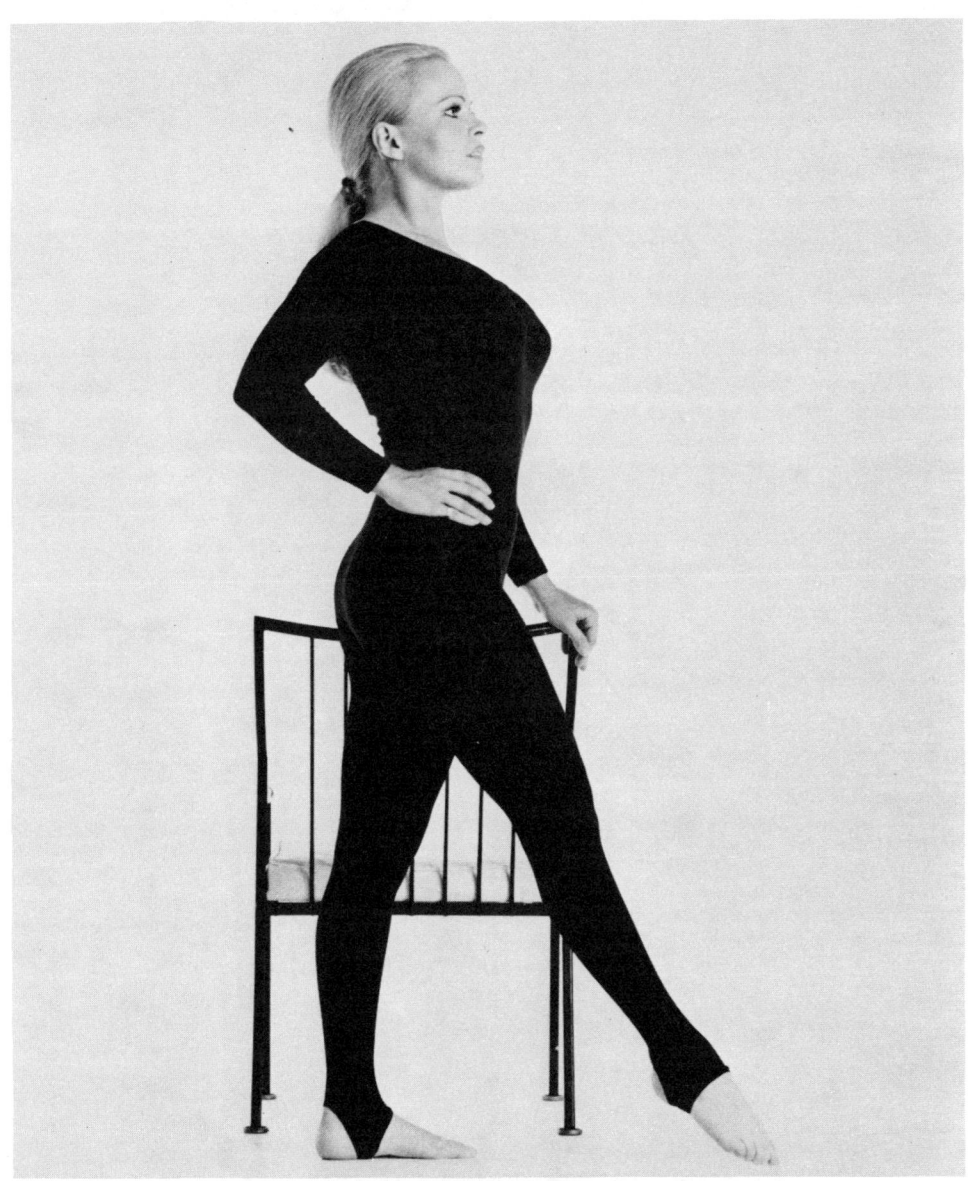

2. Knee bends. With feet together and arms extended in front of you, slowly bend your knees, then slowly stand erect again. Work up to 20 daily.

3. With your right hand on a table or counter for balance (I use the bathroom sink counter), kick your left leg as high as possible in front of you, then backward. Face the other way and kick the right leg in the same manner. Do 10 with each leg.

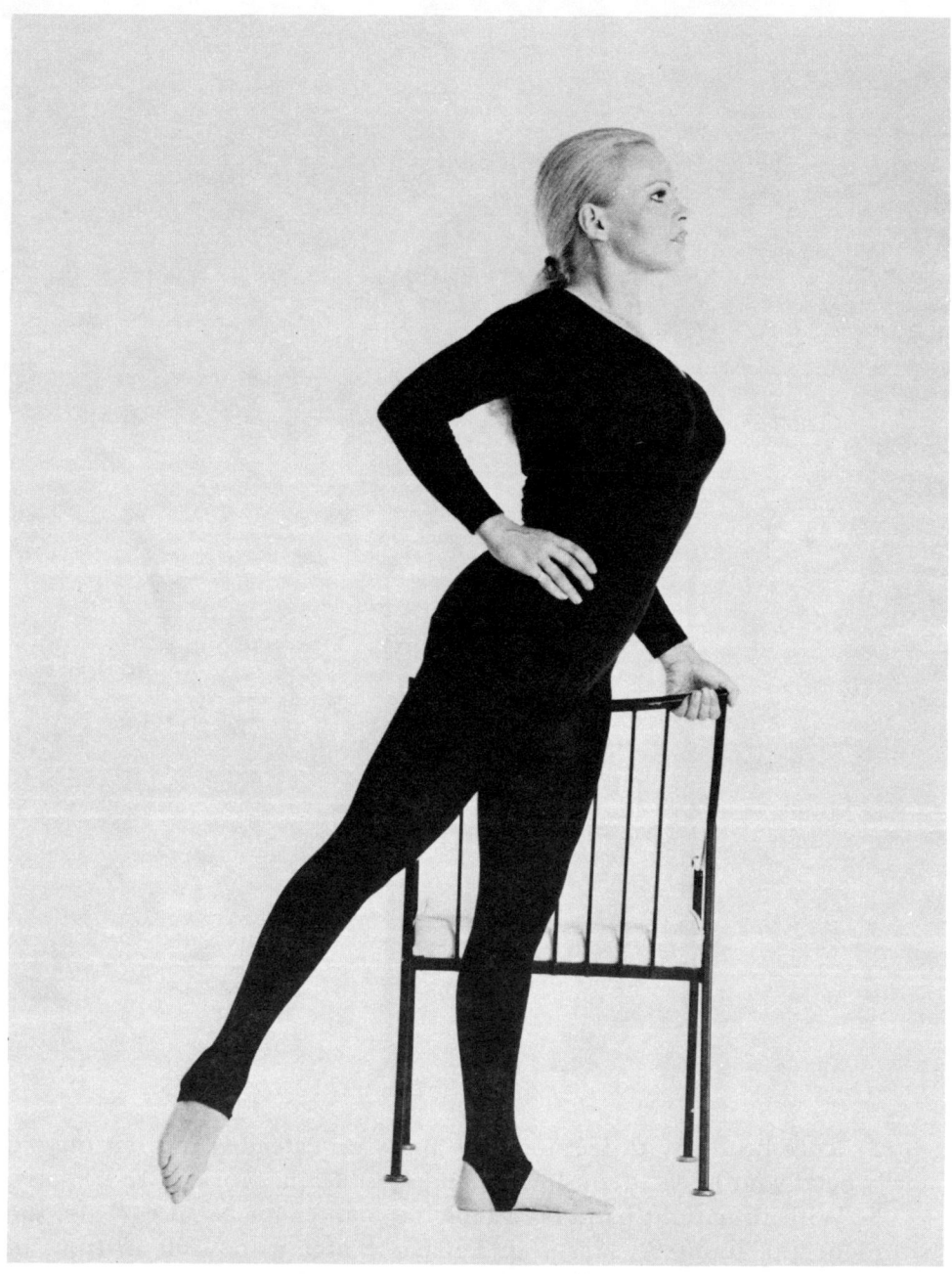

4. In the same position, using something waist high for support, swing the outer leg in front of you, toes pointed, then swing it in an arc to your side and the rear. Back and forth 10 times with each leg.

Stomach

The same as exercises 7 and 8 given in Chapter 2—sit-ups and leg raises. Begin with 3 each and gradually increase to 20. Tense the stomach muscles while doing these.

Calves

Raise on your toes, up and down. If you do this slowly, it will increase the size of your calves; if done quickly, it will decrease the size. If your balance is good, try doing this while standing on the edge of a step, heels unsupported. This gives more room for stretching the calves.

Ankles

Rotate feet from the ankles. Joyce does this frequently, as her ankles have always been weak and she needs to strengthen them for her tennis game.

Overweight Because of Thyroid Problem

Do the shoulder stand given as exercise No. 9 in Chapter 2. This brings blood to the thyroid—and the pituitary glands, brain, face, and neck. Try to include this in your daily exercise routine.

The combination of proper eating and exercise is guaranteed to establish a satisfactory weight and your top figure. The old saw that exercise makes you hungry is a fallacy; it actually decreases appetite. One more point: Joyce says we must think of it as "getting rid of" weight, not "losing." There's something psychological about losing anything, and many people are prone to attempt finding anything "lost." Just get rid of it.

You can relieve boredom by changing the order of the exercises. But please don't fail to exercise in some way, even that brisk walk around the block. Do *something!*

POSTURE

You may have a figure like a goddess, but if you don't stand straight and move well, you won't reap many second glances.

I'm guilty of bad posture—or was, for many years. My bust began to develop when I was in fifth grade; I was the second girl in my class to wear a bra. That made me different, and to a teen-ager, "being different" is a pain. It wouldn't have been so awful, maybe, if I'd sprung a decent 32B, but I kazoomed out of all proportion. I was so self-conscious that I began hunching my shoulders and crossing my arms across my chest. After a couple of years of this habit, I looked as though I was tied into a strait jacket.

My mom told me, maybe a dozen times a day, "Hold your shoulders back!" The constant admonition was a drag. Putting my shoulders back didn't do anything except make my bust stick out more. Then one day I went for a physical examination and when I walked into the doctor's office he said, "Pull up your chest."

I stared at him. "Do *what?*"

"Your chest," he said. "Lift it."

I did, and everything fantastic happened. My shoulders went back, my stomach went in, my chest went up to where it had belonged for years, and my fanny pooched forward the way models' do. What's more, all that rearrangement *felt* good.

I took to keeping it this way, because that was about the time I enrolled at the Pasadena Playhouse to study drama. At classes, I soon learned to overcome the tendency to tip my pelvis because of a slight sway back. To correct this, I squeezed the buttocks and pushed the pelvis forward—which not only helps deter back problems, but gives a longer, straighter look to the body. I stopped crossing my arms in front, and I learned to stand straight and think tall. All of which relieved pressure on internal organs by giving them the space they were meant to have.

Some years ago, I read in a magazine about a European girl who was so tall that she resorted to an extreme surgical procedure. Doctors cut two inches from her femur bones (thigh bones, the longest in the body), and I wondered what she looked like, postoperative. She might have been shorter, but she must have looked out of proportion, and probably could never wear shorts or bathing suit because of scars. Was it really worth it, to shrink two inches? I think tall is beautiful. I get a real kick when I see a tall woman standing up to her every inch of height, erect and proud. Tall women standing tall look like a million, and of course I envy them, too, because they wear clothes so beautifully. When they slump or slouch, the immediate thought is, "poor, tall girl." As a woman thinketh, so she is.

Incidentally, if you are at all self-conscious when walking toward a friend on the street or entering a room full of people, tell yourself you're a smash, and walk as if you were. If you're inordinately shy or self-conscious, you can use the gimmick employed by entertainers. No audience can make you nervous if you picture them all sitting there in their underwear. Try that one on for size sometime.

At the Playhouse, I learned how to walk. Because I'm short, I'd always taken short steps—which of course made me look shorter. I remember the day in Roland Dupre's dancing class when he singled out a short dancer. "Bobby," he told him, "you're going to have to keep your legs wider apart than the other dancers and exaggerate every arm gesture, to give the impression you're taller." I do this sometimes when walking with Bill. I start matching his steps, which not only makes me look and feel taller, but it's good for my hips.

I think the best example of learning to walk well is that of Barbara Stanwyck. Early in her career, she spent hours at the zoo, watching the big cats in their cages. If you remember Stanwyck's walk, she takes long, even strides—and the effect is marvelously fluid and graceful.

If possible, get someone to take a movie film of you while you're walking—front, back, and side views. You may discover a great deal that can be improved.

As for sitting, never plop into a chair. We film actors learn this because if we sit down in a hurry, we're likely to lower ourselves faster than the camera and disappear altogether out of its range. As models and actors learn, make sure your back is directly in front of the chair, then ease yourself down to the seat. Crossed legs, I think, are unattractive for women, as well as bad for circulation. The most graceful way you can sit is to cross your legs only at the ankles, both feet on the floor.

When getting into a car, use the same trick—back up to the seat and sit, then swing your legs into the car. Don't throw one leg in, à la John Wayne, and then haul the other after it. Exit from the car with the reverse motion—turn your body to put both feet on the ground, then stand up. If you are climbing into the back seat of a two-door car, I'm sorry to say I have no suggestions. If you can't yell, "Shotgun!" in a bid for sitting up front, you'll just have to suffer the indignity of plunging in head first with your fanny following, and then collapse into the seat. In this predicament, there is no way I know of *not* to plop.

CLOTHES

The expression, "Clothes make the man" was coined long before women's lib. Men have only to button a jacket over a paunch, and that's that. We women have a helluva lot more to deal with when choosing a wardrobe.

To begin with, when you try on clothes at a shop, do please look at your rear. Once you've decided a dress is right for you, sit down in it. There's nothing like wearing a dress for the first time and discovering it rides half way up your thighs when you sit down. I remember the dress I had made for my prom. It sported five layers of tiered scallops and looked just great during the fittings, when I was standing. The first time I sat down at the prom, all five layers rose and inverted, and each time I stood again I had to smooth each one down by hand.

On clothes and the bosom, if your bust is small, count those two blessings. Everything you wear looks great because your line is smooth. I don't understand why small-breasted women want balloons that bounce around in front of them, and create bulges that destroy any hope of looking svelte.

If you don't like your A cup, you can always wear padded bras, available at any store. Or, if you live miles from a shopping center, you can write for a catalog of super padded bras to Frederick's of Hollywood, Hollywood Boulevard, Hollywood, California.

Okay, now let's get around to big bosoms, a subject literally nearest my heart. First, wear a bra, for heaven's sake. Droopy breasts aren't attractive in the bus or at the ball. Furthermore, if you're stuck with large breasts, you are wide open to Cooper's disease, (neuralgia of the breast) an ailment that can be painful. Also, you'll have the dandy little problem of those indentations on your shoulders made by the bra straps, but at least you'll be affording support for your breasts.

If you're proud of your bosom, that's fine for you, but I'm not. And so I minimize the situation with loose clothing—sweaters, blouses, and jackets always in one size larger than normal. (I always wear tailored jackets, which make my bust appear smaller.) No horizontal stripes above the waist (in my case, none below the waist either because I'm short). And always solid colors or vertical patterns.

I'd rather cut off my nose than shop for a bathing suit. A big bosom in a bathing suit is an impossibility. A couple of years ago, manufacturers finally seemed to understand that our tops don't always match our bottoms, and put on the market mix-and-match tops and bottoms—thereby relieving me of the necessity of buying two bathing suits to get my top and my bottom properly attired for the beach. A nifty idea. But just last month I went shopping for a mix-and-match bathing suit, and every last one of the tops had padded cups. I was so infuriated I went to a rack of regular suits and bought two, one a size 7, the other an 11. I kept the 7 bottom and the 11 top, and the next day when I saw a girl at a swimming pool who had the reverse of my figure, I gave her the two remaining halves.

As for bones sticking out, that's another matter. Wide shoulders are chic, and added to that is the lovely fact that clothes *hang* well from wide shoulders. But if their width annoys you, sew the shoulder seam inward by one inch, and in blouses, a bit of puff at the shoulder helps. They did this for me at the studio when I worked in "All in the Family" because I wanted to look as small as possible. (People are usually surprised when they meet me—they say I'm thinner than they'd thought. The camera eye is myopic and spreads what it sees, so to look good on TV you must be underweight to appear normal, and if you're not, the wardrobe is planned to deceive the camera.)

If your shoulders are narrow or sloping, a simple camouflage is done with pads sewn into jacket and blouse sleeves.

Buy clothes with waistlines to match your own. If you do the exercises I've suggested for the waist, yours should tuck in where it should.

If your arms are large or flabby, adjust to the fact and hide them with sleeves. I've seen very attractive women wearing sleeveless dresses or blouses, but their flabby arms absolutely telegraphed the number of years they have been in this world.

To camouflage heavy hips, an A-line skirt is best—and at least knee length; never too short. You'll always look longer and thinner if you avoid wearing two colors—tops different than bottom—and instead choose ensembles with one color. A straight leg line in slacks as well as a nipped-in waistline in slacks and skirts will emphasize the size of hips. So instead wear wider-legged pants that drop straight down from the hip, and let your blouses hang out, to cover the hips. Above all, don't wear anything tight at the thighs, and avoid tight Levi's like a plague.

PLASTIC SURGERY

I've discussed the possibilities of plastic surgery from the neck up—now, let's lower the boom.

Bust

First, know that after you have any surgery done on the breast, it will be ten to fourteen days before you can raise your arms, to brush your hair or lift things. The aftermath includes incapacitation; you should know what it involves and plan for it.

I once took the pencil test to find out, according to a fashion magazine, if I should wear a bra. You place a pencil beneath each breast, and if they fall out, you don't need a bra. I guess I was like many women—the pencil stayed under one (one vote for a bra) and fell from the other one (one nay vote). As I've mentioned, we're all different one side from the other, and the breast that's in better condition is likely to match the hand we use most—the result of exercising the pectoral muscles on that side.

Since then, I've been casting dubious glances at my breasts and considering reduction—of both—by plastic surgery. There are two ways of doing this. The newer surgical approach is from the side, pulling sagging muscles through an incision in the arm, after which the scar is rarely visible. The other method consists of several incisions and removal of a pie-shaped wedge of breast tissue and skin. After this is removed, the nipple is recentered. Pretty heavy surgery for a woman complaining only that she has to walk pretty fast to keep from falling forward, or that she risks smothering if she stands on her head. I have to *think* about this. Is it worth it, to relieve myself of the shooting pains from the breasts' weight, the back pain, the ever-present shoulder indentations from the tug of bra straps?

Cher once told me that she has had a minor breast lift done after each baby. Her breasts enlarge with pregnancy, then sag afterward, and she's twice gone to a New York surgeon who makes a small incision and lifts the muscles, then closes her up. It works wonderfully, and you never see the scar.

People have said to me, "Sally, if you want a breast reduction or at least a lift, and you want children, why don't you wait until you've had all the babies you want?" That's what Joyce did. With each of her three pregnancies she grew bigger than Jayne Mansfield, and had enough milk for quintuplets. Her doctor always greeted her with, "How's my dairy today?" But all three boys were born prematurely and couldn't nurse because her nipples were inverted. The doctor gave her dry-up pills, after which, says Joyce, "My boobs looked like nylon stockings with nothing in them." After the last baby, she had surgery in which they went in through the chest wall, took out tissue and put in an implant. (Postoperatively, in this procedure, a woman lactates normally in future pregnancies.) This is called a mammoplasty, an enlargement of the breasts. The implant consists of silicone bags implanted under the fold of the breasts. So much progress has been made in this surgery that it's difficult to tell the difference between a normal breast and one that's had an implant.

I'm still thinking about a breast reduction, but what I'm *not* thinking about is a breast augmentation. Surgeons say these breast enlargements make for their happiest patients. Not I, said this little red hen. But for others, implants are done frequently and well. The worst that can happen is encapsulation (hardening) which occurs if the body rejects the implant. In such cases, the surgery must be performed again.

After mastectomies, many plastic surgeons will work with the thoracic surgeon to rebuild the breast postoperatively. A friend of Joyce's had both breasts removed—and replaced by plastic surgery. They look totally normal and have the same feeling to the tactile sense as normal breasts. And I know of one case in which the surgeon successfully performed the implantation within one month after the breast was removed. Joyce has reminded me to tell you that records indicate the ratio of return of malignancy is not increased by an implant.

I'm not pushing breast plastic surgery, please understand that, and I make a strong point that if you consider any of it, you must consult at least three certified plastic surgeons, plus, as I've already mentioned, talk with their prior patients.

Hip Pinch

This is removal of saddle bags from the outer thighs. Recuperative time is four to six weeks, and it most definitely leaves a scar. Which would bother you more—the bulge or the scar? Try to correct saddle bags with the exercises I've given you.

Tummy Tuck

If you've had babies and your stomach muscles are loose, no amount of exercise is going to pull skin and muscles back together. You can consider a tummy tuck. They cut at the pubic hairline, even remove the navel and replace it at the normal anatomical spot—after keeping it in a saline solution, I assure you. But a forewarning. Eventually you'll have your waistline and flat stomach returned to you, yet the interim is a long one. For fourteen days you'll have to lie flat on your back. When you finally can get up, you'll walk bent over like the hunchback of Notre Dame for six weeks. Only then will you be able to walk erect. Consider. Is it all worth it?

And remember, particularly if you are a diabetic, TELL YOUR SURGEON OF ANY AND ALL HEALTH PROBLEMS BEFORE ANY PLASTIC SURGERY IS PERFORMED.

My final contribution to this subject is Joyce's favorite reply from the plastic surgeons she has interviewed on the subject of how diet affects the outcome of plastic surgery. The doctor said, "The Coke and candy bar bunch don't heal as well."

8
Clean Smells Good

A woman can drown herself in perfume or incense and myrrh, but it availeth her nothing if she doesn't bathe.

I was surprised to learn from Joyce that the skin expels more waste than the bowels, kidneys, and lungs combined. In fact, it's possible to emit one pound of perspiration in one day. This bit of knowledge is enough in itself to force everyone into a daily bath. I can't understand why anyone would have to be *forced* to bathe. To me, a brisk shower or warm bath constitute one of the best parts of my day—a morning waker-upper and a relaxing prelude to sleep.

Bathing is downright healthy. By way of perspiration, the skin is a self-cleansing organ, but clothing inhibits the procedure, as well as prevents the skin from breathing. If impurities aren't removed by bathing, they can be reabsorbed through the skin and returned to the system. Ergo, if skin fails to function in eliminating toxic waste, this can cause a breakdown of internal organs.

People have been bathing, in a variety of ways, for a very long time. Moses commanded his people to be scrupulously clean, and bathing was included in religious rites of the Jews. David said (Psalms 51:7), "Purge me with hyssop and I shall be clean; wash me, and I shall be whiter than snow." (You can bathe in hyssop today—an aromatic mint, it is available at HFS. Put $\frac{1}{2}$ lb. in a cloth, tie securely and place it in the tub water. If you rub it gently over your body it's a wonderful cleansing and beautifying agent for the skin. You can use the bag for several baths.)

When the Roman legions went marching all over the place, the soldiers relieved their aching muscles and feet by dumping mugwort into their bath water. (Unless you look up "mugwort" in "What's THAT?" I'll bet you skip that one.)

American Indians were fond of vapor baths.

The seventeenth-century French beauty Ninon de Lenclos had men still swooning about her when she was well past seventy years old, and said that her personal fountain of youth had been her daily herb bath. Here is old Ninon's recipe: 1 handful each of dried lavendar flowers, rosemary leaves, dried mint, comfrey roots, and thyme. Mix these together in a cheesecloth bag, put this in the tub, pour boiling water to cover and let soak for 15 minutes. Then fill the tub and immerse yourself for 20 minutes. Maybe you won't be inundated by young swains, but you'll certainly smell good.

Shower or tub—choose as you wish. The shower has an advantage in that you can finish with a cold splash to close your pores . . . recommended especially if you're a city dweller. Keep a loofa in the shower; used as a massage, it will increase circulation as well as remove dry skin. (The reason people sing in the shower: According to a scientific theory of ions in the atmosphere, the negative ions affect our mood in a positive manner. Running water creates more negative than positive ions; therefore, the happy showerer. According to my own theory, the echo in a shower is so great that it makes us all feel like recording stars.)

Afterward, massage with a dry brush or towel until you feel the warmth from increased circulation. And whether shower or bath, pay attention to the fact that many toxins exit through your feet; scour them well.

In both bath and shower, avoid water that is too hot. Heat depletes energy, is weakening, and should never be used by those who are stout, or afflicted with heart problems. Joyce reminds us *never* to take a *hot* bath while fasting. On the other side of the faucet, cold water is not good for the elderly or anyone with artery disease. The warm bath is best—keep the water at your own body temperature.

Most soaps are alkaline and very drying for the skin, particularly that of the face. One soap widely advertised as pure is almost pure alkaline. Neither Joyce nor I ever use soap on our faces. For the body, we use oatmeal soap, the granules in which afford a good scrub for the skin.

How about bubble baths? Anything containing perfume, and thus alcohol, is drying to the skin. Also, some bubble bath products contain chemicals. When you are immersed in a bubble bath, remember that the vaginal area is extremely delicate, and should afterward be flushed with pure water. In point of fact, following a bubble bath, it's a good idea to rinse the entire body with pure water.

EPSOM SALT BATH

Epsom salt is great to help the skin cleanse itself. After filling the tub with water, add 2 pounds of Epsom salt and then soak in the tub for 20 minutes. After your bath, dry brush or towel massage, then oil the entire body with a vegetable oil. Never mineral oil, which inhibits the absorption of vitamin A. Read the vegetable oil label. Your skin will absorb the oil, so don't worry about staining your clothing.

OIL BATH

    1 cup of oil (corn, sesame, or olive)
    1 tbs. of good liquid shampoo
    ½ tsp. of your favorite perfume, or oil of rose geranium

Mix these in a bottle and shake well before each use. Use 2 tbs. in each bath. This does wonders for dry skin. (Caution—this makes for a slippery tub.)

HERBAL BATHS

This first one is an alternative to Mme. de Lenclos' formula. Toss a handful each of rosemary, lavendar, khus-khus roots, and rose geranium into a large pot of boiling water. To 1 part of these herbs, add 4 parts of borax crystals. Simmer for 15 minutes, strain, then add to bath water. Or use this as an after-bath rinse. Instead of adding to the bath water, you might choose to put the herbs and borax crystals into a nylon stocking and tie this to the tub faucet, letting the force of the water release the fragrance into the tub.

    For sore and aching muscles, use a bag of camomile—or mugwort.

    To relieve nervous tension, boil ½ lb. of valerian in a big pot of water for 30 minutes, then add to bath water.

    For a dry and itching skin, fill a cloth with oatmeal—½ lb. to 1 lb., depending on the amount of tub water. Tie securely and place in the water. Stay immersed for half an hour, rubbing the skin gently with the oatmeal bag.

DEODORANTS

The more properly you eat, the less body odor you will have. Odor is an indicator of your physical condition.

Before applying deodorant, close the pores by splashing under your arms with cold water, then towel dry. You don't want the chemicals in deodorant to enter your lymph glands through open pores. If you have nicked yourself while shaving, don't use deodorant until the lesion heals.

Before putting on our clothes, most of us go around with upraised arms, waiting for deodorant to dry. I used to do this until I had the bright idea of using my blow dryer, on a cool setting, to dry the armpits. You're welcome.

If you have an unpleasant and persistent body odor, you may be lacking the correct ratio of magnesium and chelated minerals. To correct this, eat a lot of greens and take 1 tsp. daily of chlorophyl, the life-giving blood of plants (available at HFS). Also at HFS, you can buy bottled sea water, which is chock full of minerals. You might put a teaspoon of this in a bottle of drinking water and keep it in the fridge.

If you have an offensive genital odor, this means a fungus or infection, and you should consult a doctor about it. To help prevent vaginal infections wear only pantyhose with a cotton crotch, and never sleep in your underwear. (Surprisingly, many people do.) You've got to allow the skin to breathe.

As a douche, baking soda is excellent. Use 1 tsp. per bag, although mix in a glass container first to avoid lumping. Or mix a light solution of comfrey tea—1 oz. to 1 qt. of water, used at body temperature. Also, a drop or two of chlorophyl is very refreshing.

SHAVING

After shaving under your arms, wait until they are completely dry before applying deodorant. As I've already mentioned, the pores can first be closed by a splash of cold water. Witch hazel will also close pores. If your underarms are irritated from shaving, use a powder deodorant.

Be careful with discarded razor blades. Wrap them *carefully* in cardboard. When my sister was a kid she bit her nails. I'll never forget the day she wanted to scratch a mosquito bite, reached into the bathroom wastebasket for a piece of paper as a tool, unknowingly picked up one wrapped around a razor blade, and gouged her thigh horribly when she scratched. Be particularly careful with used razor blades if there are children in your home.

New hair on legs is coarse and thick. If you use a depilatory here, this will "gentle" the hair, and remove it both above and below the skin surface . . . but you don't have to cream hair away every time you shave. Use of a depilatory avoids the upsetting discovery of stiff hairs poking through your nylons. If you do use a razor, slow down, and use even strokes. I can't count the times I've been at a luncheon or party and looked down to discover I'd forgotten those bits of facial tissue under my stockings, where I'd cut myself. Instead of tissue, use a styptic pencil, the sort men use for shaving nicks. And do shave slowly, even if you're in a crashing hurry to get dressed.

FRAGRANCE

There is nothing to equal good French perfume. Personally, I've found 98 per cent of other perfumes much too strong, icky, and sweet. In the morning, a strong scent is overpowering, almost nauseating. I choose to shop for men's colognes, for myself, something gentle and spicy for the daytime. I now use Bill's, and get many compliments during the day.

When the weather is warm and you need to be refreshed during the day, I'd suggest you carry in your purse a plastic bottle of astringent or freshener, such as Sea Breeze, and periodically apply it at your pulse points with a cotton ball. Another good spot is the back of your neck. When I'm working and go backstage between acts, some kind soul is always there with a towel soaked in Sea Breeze and pats it all over me during costume change. It's refreshing, it closes the pores, and has a nice fragrance.

If you shower or bathe in the mornings, you can combine any natural oil—almond, avocado, sesame oil—with a drop of light perfume, and rub this gently over your body. Don't grease yourself, but use it sparingly—and as I've promised, your skin will absorb it before your clothes make contact.

In the evenings, of course, you can turn a lot sexier, but please do keep away from strong and sweet perfumes, and find one that you feel suits you. I hope it isn't musk oil. I once had to leave a dinner unfinished because the waitress left a trail of heavy musk scent that smelled like something washed up on a beach.

TEETH

No matter how hard you brush your teeth, you never totally remove food particles that are stuck between them. This is one of the major causes of mouth odor. Dental tape (not floss) should do the trick, and should be used before you go to bed. This prevents decay during the night, and also if you've drawn a little blood, gives your gums time to heal overnight.

Watch your intake of milk. Milk is lactic acid and destroys teeth. That's why nature gives us two sets of teeth—the first for the milk-drinking years. The new set doesn't stand up well under the continued onslaught of lactic acid. Even primitive societies know better—adults don't drink milk. In our own society, milk sold commercially is processed with formaldehyde in order to lengthen its shelf life. One more reason not to drink too much of it. If you're a milk buff, drink *certified* raw milk.

The best toothpaste you can use is a mixture of baking soda and salt —2 parts baking soda to 1 part salt. Wet your brush, dip often into the mixture and brush vigorously. This not only cleans your teeth, but also removes tartar and is great for the gums.

A mouthwash that is available to everyone—salt and warm water. Particularly before retiring.

ADDENDA

I trust I don't have to caution you, once you're clean as the driven snow, to wear clean clothes. It's a simple matter these days; we no longer have to go down to the river and scrub soiled laundry on rocks. There's no excuse for unclean clothing.

Also, while I doubt that one out of a thousand of you ever uses body makeup, I think I ought to give a tip for removing it. I once did a film for which my entire body was covered with makeup, except for underpants and bra areas. Even before they finished applying it, I began worrying about rubbing the stuff *in* when I bathed later. My makeup man told me to take a cool shower—so that I could wash it off with closed pores—and *then* take a hot shower. The same goes for your facial makeup; if you're going to use soap and water, use cool water first.

9
Hands Up and Feet Forward

The human hand is a wondrous mechanism of nineteen bones. According to anthropology, it has been largely responsible for man's advance beyond other creatures. The hand can build a house, sew a quilt, scratch a back, climb a cliff, bake a cake, and adjust a microscope. It is often taken for granted and unappreciated until it becomes inoperative because of a bandage or cast. Hands are not only functional—they are, or can be, beautiful.

Many people, particularly nervous Nellies, never know what to *do* with their hands. If you are of Latin extraction and given to gestures, that's your nature, but it is so attractive to see people who keep their hands in repose. When you are sitting, you'll have the look of serenity if you keep your hands in your lap, one in the palm of the other. Actors have a terrible time with their hands. Cigarettes were always a good prop to clutch at, but these days you see very few actors smoking on screen. Ronald Colman had the pockets of all suits worn for roles sewn shut. He said that without pockets to stuff his hands into, he *had* to learn what to do with them.

So keep your hands still and in your lap when sitting—and keep them away from your face. Teen-agers are particularly guilty on this score, forever fussing with their hair and face. You know now what that germy habit does to facial skin, and there's an additional tabu for those who are allergic to nail polish. Many of us are. Joyce has discovered this allergy in more than one of her clients who complain of itching eyes and have a habit of rubbing them, replete with nail polish.

The one gesture I can't abide, a purely personal repugnance, is the extension of the little finger. I don't know where the idea originated that sticking out a pinky is dainty. To me, it looks like an antenna looking for a radio wave, and when Bill does it, I reach over and shove the finger back next to the others.

Another pet hate of mine is a limp handshake. I don't think there's anything more unsettling than a dead-fish handshake, from women as well as men. I find I tend to dislike that person immediately. There's no warmth, no sincerity. If you ever meet me, do please grasp my hand firmly and shake hands a bit—mute but solid evidence that you're happy to meet me, not bored stiff.

Hands show age sooner than most parts of the body, so it's important to begin taking care of them while you're young. If you're no longer young, start now. It's never too late to begin taking care of yourself.

First of all, watch out for detergents. You wouldn't put a soap detergent on your face, so why do you dip your hands into it? I know, you may have to clean the house, but you can buy a package of disposable gloves to wear while you're scrubbing. You can use the same pair over and over again, and they are quite reasonably priced. If you do expose your hands to the alkaline properties in household cleaners, neutralize this afterward by rinsing your hands in apple cider vinegar. Or rub them with the juice of a lemon.

If your hands are already red and worn looking, take protein and calcium internally. This will not cure the condition, as alkaline destroys faster than it is possible to repair from the inside, but it may well help.

When you apply moisturizer to your face, remember to use it on your hands, too.

Here's the best formula I know of to nourish the hands. I'm sure most of you have at some time gone to bed wearing gloves to cover creamed hands for the night. Try this one, with cotton gloves, and you'll be pleasantly surprised.

HAND-NOURISHING TREATMENT

4 tbs. honey
4 tbs. almond oil
2 tbs. lecithin granules
1 egg yolk

Warm the honey in a small pan over a low flame. Remove pan from the heat and blend in the oil and lecithin. Let cool before adding the egg yolk, then blend well.

FINGERNAILS

I hope you don't bite them; it's a difficult habit to overcome. That sister of mine who bit her nails was finally cured when our father hypnotized her, but chances are small that you live with a hypnotist.

So, assuming you have nails, keep them clean.

If your nails are marred by ridges, this may be due to a prior injury. If not, it's likely a thyroid problem. For this, do your shoulder stand every day, bringing blood to the thyroid.

For nails that are thin, soak them in gelatin for 15 minutes every day. Taken internally, gelatin is reputed to be good for nails. Not true. Gelatin is an incomplete protein. Thin nails may be due to a lack of calcium, or improper diet. So, again, make sure your diet is balanced, and take the full quota of calcium lactate, 1,200 mg. daily.

To find a good nail cream, read labels and choose one that contains vitamins A, D, E, and B, as well as pantothenic acid (which might be termed on the label as panthenol). The B vitamins are important. Brewers' yeast is loaded with B vitamins, so if you're drinking your skin shake, you're feeding your nails.

Nails don't have to be long to look good. Always file them in one direction, not back and forth as if sawing a log. Filing in the same direction leaves nails stronger. Don't file them to a point. Instead, square them off a bit, and they won't break as easily.

You really should have a manicure every other week, and it's quite simple to do this yourself. First, soak the nails in a bowl of water with gentle soap suds (*not* detergent), then push back the cuticle with a towel or orange stick.

As for polish, the first step, of course, is to remove the old polish properly. The worst thing you can do to nails is peel off the polish, a nervous habit that eventually will create ridges. Remove it completely from both nail and cuticle with polish remover. This is very drying, so after its use, oil the cuticles with olive or wheat-germ oil. Or vitamin E squeezed from a capsule.

Some women cannot wear polish without their nails going into a three-month decline. If this is true in your case, just don't use it. Instead, buff your nails; they'll be just as attractive. After all, polish is not mandatory for lovely nails. Besides, it's caustic, therefore an irritant.

If you wear polish, this is one more reason to keep your hands away from your face.

FEET

Feet are just as much of an engineering miracle as hands. They have the same structure, yet give the added service of bearing your weight. In an average lifetime they carry you a distance equal to three times around the world.

Despite this burden, they are sensitive things. Many nerve endings are in our feet . . . a good reason why you've so often heard people say, "When my feet hurt, I hurt all over."

Feet are the most neglected part of our anatomy. The poor soles are the recipient of all rejected poisons from the system, which cling firmly to the bottom of the feet, coating the pores. It isn't the shoes that cause foot odor, it's the feet themselves, and the reason is they are not kept properly clean.

A fine foot soak is made with oat straw, available at a HFS. Pour boiling water over 4 handfuls and let steep for 10 minutes. Then add cooler water until you have a comfortable temperature. This is marvelous for tired feet.

Another refresher is the mixture of rubbing alcohol with a bit of oil of wintergreen. You can add to this 1 tsp. of chlorophyl and some aloe vera.

A simpler foot bath is that old standby, Epsom salt, which not only soothes the feet, but softens corns and calluses.

Before attacking a callus, soften it with olive oil, or the same cream you use on your face. Then use your pumice stone. You should keep one of these in your bathroom to be used daily after your bath. With pumicing, a callus will eventually disappear. Another good foot tool is a hindu stone, available at the drug store. Use this around and under the toenails to remove dead cuticle.

After you've used pumice and hindu stone, try the following treatment for removing corns and callus altogether. Place over the trouble spots a piece of lemon peel with some pulp attached, bandage, and wear to bed. Remove in the morning. After five nights of this procedure, you should be able to peel off the offending corn and callus. (Those of you who saw the movie *Funny Lady* might remember the scene where Barbra Streisand rubbed her elbows and feet with lemon before going to bed. It seemed silly to Jimmy Caan and perhaps you, too, but now you know why.)

If you are troubled by athlete's foot, apply cider vinegar to the areas, frequently. This is touted to be effective, although I'm happy to say I haven't yet had reason to try it.

Go barefoot around the house. Feet are seldom permitted to breathe, encased in shoes and stockings all day, so let them be free as often as possible. Not in public—city streets are the best place to pick up foot disease via a disgusting amount of dirt. In addition, walking on cement toughens the soles, thereby creating more work for the feet to expel impurities. Your home or lawn—nothing like the feel of grass on bare feet—are recommended.

Prop up your feet as often as possible—simple to do when you're reading or watching television. This relieves pressure on the veins.

Also when you're sitting, take time to rub your feet, exerting gentle pressure at the arch and ball of the feet. This is wondrously relaxing, as well as beneficial.

When Joyce gives a facial, she always massages the feet and hands with the same moisturizer she uses on the face. She encloses both hands and feet in plastic bags, then puts them in heated booties and mittens for the 90 minutes it takes to give the facial. You can do the same by putting hands and feet in gloves and heavy socks after you've soaked them in cream. Leave them on for about an hour—overnight is even better. You won't believe the change in skin texture. You really ought to give your hands and feet this treat once a week.

SIMPLE FOOT EXERCISES

1. After your bath, stand on one end of a bath towel and try to rake the rest of the towel toward you.

2. In bare feet, try picking up a pencil, marble, a spool of thread, any small object, with your toes. This limbers the arches as well as exercising the rest of the feet.

Let's leave feet for a minute, and talk about your legs. If your legs are heavy, wear dark-colored stockings. If too thin, wear light colors. Enhance or detract, depending on the way you score your legs, by skirt length. Pantsuits cover a multitude of leg problems. As for myself, I wear support hose. They used to be horrors, and *looked* like support hose, but today you can't tell the difference. I'm on my feet a great deal in my work, and I find this support most helpful in relieving tired legs. If you are pregnant, you most definitely should wear support hose—the control type that holds you in almost as well as a girdle. An ounce of prevention is worth a pound of varicose veins, which, if you care to know, are created by constipation and the resultant strain of elimination, plus the constant pressure endured by the legs in standing or walking.

Back to your feet and your toenails. Feet have nails, too, and they should be given the same care as your fingernails. In addition to the hindu stone, give the cuticle frequent applications of cream or oil, and push it back the same way you do fingernail cuticle.

When cutting toenails, cut them straight across. Pointed toenails lead to ingrown nails—at the very least they'll tear holes in your stockings.

The one problem your heroic feet never have to undergo is biting. If you bite your toenails, more power to you.

10
Voice Vibes

As Ma Bell says, your voice is *you*. Much like your eyes, the voice is a mirror to your soul, personality, mood, opinion of yourself, and of the person to whom you are speaking.

Most people don't pay nearly enough attention to their own voices. Unless you have heard yourself as others hear you, you don't know how your voice actually sounds. This is because the head and mouth become echo chambers for your voice, which only *you* hear from the inside where it's created as well as the sound waves from the air surrounding you.

The only way to hear your true voice is to listen to yourself on tape. If you've already done this, you know about the shock. If you haven't, you're in for a surprise and will, like everyone else, say, "That's not what I sound like, is it?"

But it is. And 99 per cent of voices can be improved in several ways.

The first is diction. Americans tend to talk much too fast, slurring their words. Today's teen-agers are the worst culprits. I don't know why "today's," but it's a fact that they mumble and run their words together until their speech is unintelligible. "Jeet?" means that one teen has just asked another, "Did you eat?" Another example: "Wyjadwit" is translated as, "Why did you do it?" Diction has gone out the door.

Come on, kids. Language is the soul and foundation of civilization, and you're stamping it out.

Once you've listened to yourself on tape—preferably by recording a normal conversation with a friend, during which you should try to ignore the running tape—I trust you'll want to improve your diction. It's simple to learn—enunciation is accomplished by opening the mouth and using the jaw. Cut a small piece of paper into a pie-shaped wedge. Face a mirror, and do the exercise taught actors. Say the "ah" sound, preceded by consonants. Bah, cah, dah, fah, gah, etc. If you can't insert the point of the paper into your mouth while you're making these sounds, you're not opening your mouth wide enough. If you'll do this every day for a few minutes, you'll soon notice that people have ceased asking you to repeat what you've just said. It's a nuisance to have to ask others to repeat; it always makes me feel that people think I have a hearing problem, which I don't.

The second thing you should note when listening to your voice is the timbre. Some people who speak loudly have a resonance that carries a great distance, others merely talk too darned loud. I'm sure you, too, have had a restaurant dinner hour disturbed by someone in the next booth who shouts his conversation. Yelling is not only offensive, it's the wrong way to get attention. I think it was Greta Garbo who said that the secret of getting attention is a soft voice. A friend of mine studied at the Royal Academy in London and has one of the softest voices I've ever heard. People absolutely lean toward him to catch what he's saying, and he's always in command of a group conversation. So, if you tend to shout your thoughts to the neighborhood, concentrate on lowering your volume. You may not be *aware* your voice is too loud, but if others have been asking you to keep it down or you can remember friends shushing you, you're probably guilty of too much volume.

Thirdly, the tone of your voice. Is it too low, harsh, raspy? Is it thin, squeaky, too high? You can change it, I promise you. You can do it to some extent by *thinking* about it, but it would be well worth the trouble to take lessons from a vocal or singing teacher. You don't have to study opera; most teachers will be glad to give you only a couple of lessons, including voice exercises that will lower or raise the pitch of your voice.

Vocal cords are like two rubber bands. As you speak, air goes through them and they vibrate, rubbing against each other. A low sound makes them vibrate slowly, with a high pitch they stretch tighter, grow thinner, and vibrate faster. Most everyone has a lower voice upon wakening because the cords have been rested, and as the day goes on with its attendant tensions, the voice becomes higher. (You might tape yourself morning and evening to illustrate this point.) You can raise or lower it permanently by exercising, perhaps with a piano, merely using a syllable (such as me-me-me), working upward in scale to make the voice higher, or downward to make it lower.

I've learned a lot about my own voice. When I moved away from home and began answering my own phone, people calling me would say, "Is your mother there?" When I realized my voice was childlike—a truly unfortunate pitch because it lacks authority—I went to work and lowered it. At the Pasadena Playhouse, I almost failed in the subject of voice because I had a problem the teacher called glottic shock. This meant I forced too much air through my vocal cords when speaking, so that I was actually burping air rather than pushing it through smoothly. The result was that I sounded hoarse, as though I was getting a cold. They taught me diaphragm breathing, which all singers learn. This is breathing from the diaphragm, rather than the throat. Watch yourself in a mirror as you breathe. If your chest and/or shoulders heave, you are breathing shallowly—and speaking through your throat. Then lie on your back, a position in which all of us breathe properly, through the diaphragm. If you put your hands on your lower ribs, you'll feel the diaphragm expanding and contracting. When air comes from way down there, going up through your throat as through a long stovepipe, the voice is more resonant, richer, warmer. If you go to a vocal coach, he or she will teach you how to practice proper breathing until you do it involuntarily.

Take care of your voice. Misuse through shouting and screaming can permanently injure the vocal cords, and often will create nodes, which may need to be removed surgically. If your voice has changed recently and become raspy, it would be a good idea to see an ENT (ear, nose, throat) doctor and have your cords checked out.

Although actors are taught to project their voices without damaging the vocal cords, they nevertheless often get what is called "Vegas throat." I got through my own Las Vegas act because I was in a club with a good sound system where I was able to hear my voice over the sound of the band, and therefore didn't have to yell to hear myself. But I blew it in San Francisco, where the room's sound system was bad. After three nights I lost my voice and had to rest two days, then when I returned to the stage the following night I hurt the vocal cords so badly I was sent to an ENT, who prescribed total silence for two weeks, not even a whisper. Good-bye to my second week in San Francisco.

Laughing, too, can injure your voice. I know there's nothing more enjoyable than a good laugh, throwing back your head and letting go, but if done incorrectly, it's dangerous. At a singing lesson one day I missed three notes in the middle of my range, and my teacher asked what I'd done to my voice. I remembered then that that same morning I had screamed with laughter. After that, I tried to cultivate a soft, almost soundless laugh . . . more of a giggle than a roar.

Another thing your voice tells others is your attitude toward them. Telephone operators are taught pleasant voices by practicing speaking before a mirror, with a smile on their faces. This carries through into the tone of the voice, and you'll get a lot more service from people on the other end of a phone if you sound pleasant rather than hostile. So put a smile into your voice.

Take a few lessons if you can, and learn corrective exercises. If you can't, work on your voice by yourself. Try to sound like a Shakespearean actor during your solo sessions, and you'll find that your public voice will improve. Everybody can do it, and it's fun. In no time, you'll be speaking in pearl-shaped tones and, for a change, people will understand what you say.

11
What's THAT

All about herbs, spices, and things you've read in this book that sounded foreign to you. I think you'll find it interesting, and certainly helpful. For those of you who are unacquainted with this whole new world of natural products, it is an excellent reference, written by Joyce herself. And for those who've already delved into the subject, it is a font of information, much of which might still be new to you.

You can buy these products at drug stores if they are followed by the code letters (DS). Most of them are available at health food stores, identified by (HFS). If there is no such shop in your town or neighborhood, you can get them from firms called herbal houses; code letters (HH). At the end of this chapter you'll find a list of (HH) sources throughout the nation, from which you can order by mail.

Agar-Agar   (HFS, HH)
A seaweed containing glose, a powerful gelatinizing agent. Glose is a carbohydrate widely used to correct constipation. Agar-Agar is boiled in water, forming the mucilage you will use.

Aloe vera   (HFS, HH)
A succulent plant in the leaves of which is a mucilaginous substance that has an almost instantaneous healing affect when applied to burns, insect bites, and inflammations. Legend says aloe is the only plant that grew in the Garden of Eden still available to us. The Indians call it "wand of heaven" because of its medicinal powers. It cures wounds, ulcers, heat rash, and

poison ivy. You need only apply the cool, gummy juice direct from the fresh leaves.

Aveeno   (HFS, HH, DS)

A commercial oatmeal preparation for bathing.

Basil   (HFS, GROCERY)

From your spice shelf, basil stimulates hair growth, is good for split ends, and has a nice fragrance.

Burdock Root   (HFS, HH)

Conditions, cleans, and heals the scalp. Burdock is one of the best blood purifiers known. A tea is made with 1 oz. of chopped burdock root to 1½ pts. of water. It is a good wash for boils, ulcers, and scaly skin disorders. Taken alone, or in combination with yellow dock and sarsparilla, it has been found to be a cure for eczema. Burdock is an alternative—which means it works a gradual restoration of healthy functioning of all internal organs.

Camomile   (HFS, HH)

As a relaxant, drink camomile tea with lemon and honey at bedtime. Brew the tea with 1 oz. of camomile to 8 oz. of water, in a covered pan so that the medicinal value is not lost in evaporation. Fine for control of dandruff. Makes hair shine, heals irritated and/or dry scalp. For a hair rinse, put a handful each of camomile and rosemary into 1 qt. of water and bring to a boil. Simmer, covered, for 3 minutes. Remove, steep for 3 hours, and strain. Pour out the required quantity for scalp and hair massage every night, then rinse thoroughly with water. This will tone the hair, set it, and improve the color for blondes and redheads. The Egyptians revered camomile for its curative powers.

Celandine   (HFS, HH)

A plant used as a drug since the Middle Ages. The parts we use are the whole herb, dried—or the fresh juice of the plant. It's not to be taken internally, but has great medicinal value for eczema, scaly skin, ringworms, and corns. For warts, the raw juice is pressed from the main stems and rubbed directly on the wart. Russian researchers claim celandine has been effective in cancer cases. The plant called greater celandine is referred to here; lesser celandine is a flower.

Chelation   (HFS)

The mechanism that furnishes reactions which make possible the interrelated functioning of vitamins, amino acids, minerals, and hormones. Functioning of our bodies depends on the chelation process. When a mineral is chelated, this protects the mineral in a stable organic product. Chelation is also essential for the formation of the enzyme systems that control the body's metabolism.

Cholesterol

Despite the trouble it can cause, cholesterol is vital to body function. It helps in the formation of vitamin D, the bile salts, and both the sex and adrenal hormones. The body manufactures its own cholesterol, and neither this nor the cholesterol obtained from NATURAL foods causes deposits in the arteries. It's the cholesterol in processed foods that can be dangerous. In its natural state, cholesterol is accompanied by lecithin, a cholesterol emulsifier. (See Lecithin.)

Clover   (HFS, HH)

Clover is valuable in healing sores, and is a good cleansing herb. It can be added to salves and applied topically as an added healing agent. In Russia, red clover is prized by herbalists as a "God given remedy for cancer." White clover has no known results in cancer treatment.

Comfrey   (HFS, HH)

An astringent that removes moisture and retains natural oils. Very nutritious, it is good for dry hair and scalp. Both the root and leaves are used. In the Middle Ages, people grew it for use in healing broken bones; they called it "knit bone." Used as a poultice, it is very healing for cuts, burns, ulcers, swelling, any type of skin or scalp problem. Use 1 oz. to one pt. of water, boil 30 minutes, and strain.

Elderflower (HFS, HH)

Only the blossoms should be used in making elderflower water, which is an official preparation of the British Pharmacopoeia. This is excellent for cleansing the skin, bleaching freckles, and soothing a sunburn. Fill a large jar with elderflower blossoms, press them down, then pour 2 qts. of boiling water over them. Cool, strain, and refrigerate. For oily skin, add 1½ oz. of alcohol or witch hazel. (The odor at first will be disagreeable, but with time becomes aromatic.)

Eyebright (HFS, HH)

An herb reputed to strengthen the eyes when applied topically. It is usually combined with golden seal tea, which has antibiotic properties. Boil ½ oz. of each in 8 oz. of water, let cool. It can be infused with milk instead of water before application to the eyes, which can be done both externally and as eyedrops. Fine for itching, irritated eyes.

Golden Seal (HFS, HH)

American Indians used the root of this plant as a tonic for stomach problems, sore eyes, and general ulceration. It is a remedy for indigestion; also has a healing affect on mucous membranes. Make a tea, using 1 oz. of the root to one pt. of water, boil 30 minutes, and strain. The generic name of Golden Seal is Hydrastis—injections of Hydrastine are helpful for inflammation of the colon and rectum.

Henna (HFS, HH)

Flowers, powdered leaves. Henna not only tints the hair but gives it body. It is extremely penetrative and a very effective dye, but its one fault as a dye is its astringency. After henna applications, a bland oil such as sunflower or corn oil should be rubbed into the hair.

Kefir (HFS, GROCERY, DAIRY)

Kefir is a liquid yoghurt. You can make your own with kefir grains, which you can get by mail from the R. A. J. Biological Laboratory, 35 Park Avenue, Blue Point, Long Island, New York. Your grocery might have it; my own is delivered by my milkman. Stir 1 tbs. of kefir grains into a glass of milk and allow to stand at room temperature overnight. When the milk coagulates, it's ready to eat. Strain it to save the grains for the next batch. You can make a kefir shake by putting it into a blender with fresh fruit—it's particularly good with strawberries. Kefir is also great on salads. It's eaten by Eastern Europeans, those renowned centenarians who seem to live forever.

Khus Khus   (HFS, HH)

Aromatic roots of khus khus are a favorite in the West Indies, where dried roots are placed in drawers as insect repellents, and at the same time give delicate fragrance to clothing.

Lanolin   (DS, COSMETIC COUNTERS)

Wool fat, made from a coating found on sheep's wool. When mixed with water, lanolin forms an emulsion. This fat is closely related to the natural secretions of human beings and is excellent for very dry skin.

Lavendar Flowers   (HFS, HH)

Good for split ends. Prepare by pouring boiling water over the flowers and steeping for 10 minutes until the aroma is released. Lavendar flowers were used in times gone by as a condiment and for flavoring foods. A few drops of the essence of lavendar in a hot foot bath will relieve fatigue.

Lecithin   (HFS, DS)

Necessary because it emulsifies cholesterol. That is to say, lecithin breaks down cholesterol into small particles that move easily in the blood stream and are absorbed as needed by tissues. Lecithin is found in egg yolk, soy beans, cereal, nuts and seeds, and the oils of corn, soy, sunflower, and wheat germ. 1 tbs. of soy oil daily constitutes a protective supply. (See Cholesterol.)

Lemon

The parts used are the rind, juice, and oil. Grate the rind and squeeze the juice, then use 1 part lemon to 3 parts water. This is a fine astringent and is used as a lotion for sunburn, eczema, and burns. It's also good for ringworms and any type of scaly skin or scalp.

Lemon Grass (HFS, HH)

Rich in vitamin A. A conditioner good for both oily hair and dandruff. It has astringent qualities, is nutritious, and has a nice fragrance.

Loofa (HFS, DS)

A sponge made from the fibrous interior of the dried fruit from the luffa plant. A wonderful body scrub in your shower or bath, but too rough to use on your face.

Mugwort (HFS, HH)

The name stems from the fact that mugwort was used to flavor beer before the introduction of hops. In past centuries, it was believed to prevent sunstroke, fatigue, and even evil spirits. Mugwort contains tannin, and is valuable as an astringent. It's good for the stomach; has diuretic properties. If mixed with honey to make a poultice, it will remove the marks of a bruise.

Nettle (HFS, HH)

A conditioner that makes hair shine, stimulates growth, and aids in a dandruff problem. Both the herb and seeds are used. Simmer a handful of young nettles in 1 qt. of water for 2 hours, strain and bottle when cold. To prevent falling hair, and to make hair soft and glossy, massage the scalp with this lotion every other night. For stimulating hair growth, the old herbalists recommended combing the hair daily with nettle juice. They suggested 1 oz. of herb to 8 oz. of water. A good hair lotion can also be prepared by boiling the entire plant in vinegar and water, then straining and adding your favorite cologne. The tea of nettle is a corrective for rashes, eczema, and dandruff. No green vegetable excels the nettle in mineral and vitamin content. Nettle is rich in chlorophyl. Nettle juice can be made in a juicer.

Onion Leaves (GROCERY)

Buy from the spice shelf, or if available, use leaves from fresh onion. Onion leaves are excellent for inducing hair growth. To remove brown spots from the skin, mix ½ tsp. of onion juice with 1 tsp. cider vinegar and use as a wash. As a treatment for baldness, provided hair roots are still alive, use 1 part of onion mixed with 10 parts of unrefined cod liver oil and 5 parts of raw egg yolk. This should be beaten thoroughly and applied to the scalp once a week.

Papaya Leaves   (HFS, HH, GROCERY)

The juice is used to remove freckles. Leaves are used as a substitute for soap. When the unripe fruit itself is pierced, a milky juice is collected in a basin and allowed to gel. This is called papain. Papain is dried in the sun, and is an aid to digestion. Leaves are used for healing sores, boils, and ulceration.

Peach Leaves   (HFS, HH, PEACH TREE)

The usual decoction of 1–8 oz. of water is good for open sores, warts, and irritations. It is stimulating to hair growth and healing to the scalp.

Provitamin

Any food substance that changes into a vitamin when ingested.

Quassia Bark   (HFS, HH)

Good for dandruff or oily hair, a fine conditioner, and effective in removing hair insects. Quassia bark contains quassin, pectin, volatile oil, sulphate of lime. For a hair rinse, use a tea made by using 1 oz. of chopped quassia bark to 1 pt. of water. Boil for 15 minutes and let cool.

Rosebuds   (HFS, ROSE BUSH)

Good for oily hair and dandruff, plus its fragrance.

Rosemary   (HFS, HH)

A conditioner that should be in every hair rinse. It's good for split ends, heals the scalp, stimulates growth, makes hair shine, and has a lovely fragrance. The ancients said that rosemary strengthened the memory. We use it for tonic action and its astringent qualities. It stimulates hair bulbs to renewed activity and prevents premature baldness. One of the best hair rinses known, preventing dry scalp and dandruff, is made by using both leaves and flowers of the dried plant and boiling a handful of each with 1 oz. of borax. (Strain, and use when cooled.) To make the hair glossy, mix well 2 oz. of rosemary, 1 oz. of raspberry leaves, and 2 oz. of red sage. Place a handful in a small bowl and fill with boiling water. Cover and let stand until cold, then strain. This solution is brushed into the hair once or twice daily. The concoction should be made every day, as it does not keep. Mexicans use rosemary as a treatment for falling hair. They mash 20 grams of the herb and steep in pure alcohol for one week, then massage the scalp with the solution twice a day.

Southernwood   (HFS, HH)

The herb has antiseptic properties, and as a hair rinse is beneficial for diseases of the scalp and scalp parasites. For a hair rinse, use 2 oz. to 1 pt. of water and steep for 20 minutes. For a scalp massage, mix a little olive oil into the rinse.

Tannin

Encourages natural oils to remain in the hair, also aids in correcting dandruff. Tannin is present in camomile, wild cherry bark, and most teas and herbs.

Theobromine   (DS)

A crystaline alkaloid prepared from the dried seed of a plant, or made synthetically from xanthine. Its properties are similar to those of caffeine. It is used as a diuretic and muscle relaxant.

Valerian   (HFS, HH)

Lessens pain, promotes sleep, is an antispasmodic, yet has none of the side affects of narcotics. It is sometimes called All Heal. The fresh root is more powerful than the dried root. Steep 1 oz. of either in 8 oz. of hot water. Do not boil.

Wild Cherry   (HFS, HH)

The bark and branches are used medicinally as a tonic and astringent. Herbal houses will supply either leaves or bark. Wild cherry bark contains starch, resin, tannin, gallic acid, lignin, salts of calcium potassium, iron, and a volatile oil.

Willow Bark (HFS, HH)

Cleans, conditions, stimulates hair growth, heals abraised scalp. A great skin and scalp tonic is made by boiling 1 oz. of bark to each 8 oz. of water for 30 minutes, then strain. Good astringent qualities and natural antibiotic properties.

Yarrow (HFS, HH)

The whole herb is used in the decoction—1 oz. of the herb to 8 each oz. of water. It is astringent, tonic, mildly aromatic, and healing. Said to be a preventative for baldness if the scalp is washed with it.

Yellow Dock (HFS, HH)

An herb helpful for dry skin and scalp. Boil 1 oz. of the root in 8 oz. of vinegar until the fiber is softened, then mix the pulp with a bland skin ointment such as Vaseline, to accelerate the healing effect.

SOURCES FOR INGREDIENTS

(if a health food store is unavailable)

Arizona:	International Academy of Biological Medicine P. O. Box 31313 Phoenix, AR 85046
California:	Herb Products Co. 11012 Magnolia Boulevard North Hollywood, CA 91601
	Herbs of the World Co. P. O. Box 4100 Pasadena, CA 91106
	Nature's Herb Co. 281 Ellis Street San Francisco, CA 94102
Illinois:	Calumet Herb Co. P. O. Box 248 So. Holland, IL 60473

Indiana:	Indiana Botanic Gardens P. O. Box 5 Hammond, IN 46325
Michigan:	Harvest Health, Inc. 1944 Eastern Avenue S.E. Grand Rapids, MI 49507
New York:	Franklin Chemists 764 Franklin Avenue Brooklyn, NY
	Kiel Pharmacy, Inc. 109 Third Avenue New York, NY 10003
Pennsylvania:	Haussmann's Pharmacy, Inc. 534–536 Girard Avenue Philadelphia, PA 19123
	Penn Herb Co. 603 North Second Street Philadelphia, PA 19123
CANADA:	Dominion Herb Distributors, Inc. 61 St. Catherine Street West Montreal 18, Quebec, Canada

12

Joyce Virtue on Vitamins and Minerals

VITAMINS

Vitamins are commonly thought to be stimulants. This is a misconception. Vitamins are chemical substances that act as catalysts in body processes, helping to create energy through oxidation of protein, fats, and carbohydrates. Vitamins are organic food substances; i.e., substances existing only in living plants or animals. In foods, they exist in minute quantities. Plants manufacture their own vitamins, and animals obtain theirs from plants or the ingestion of herbivorous animals.

Vitamins are not foods in the sense of carbohydrates, fats, and proteins. These three are broken down into other substances, which the body uses in the process of metabolism. Not so with vitamins, which retain their original form in the body and are built into body structure, where they are important parts of the working of all cells. By their mere presence in the cells, they bring about certain changes . . . the reason they are called catalysts.

In this natural process, vitamins are not destroyed—but unfortunately they *can* be removed by specific agents taken into the body via the digestive system.

In the case of trace minerals—iodine, for instance—the presence or absence of vitamins in very small amounts means the difference between being sick or well.

Basically, there are two different kinds of vitamins—those that can be dissolved in fats, and those that dissolve in water. Vitamins A, D, and E, found in liver and eggs, are fat soluble and are retained in the liver. The water-soluble vitamins, B complex and C, are found in fruits and vegetables and are not retained in the body but are eliminated. Therefore, the body's needs for water-soluble vitamins is constant.

In a U. S. Department of Agriculture survey of 6,000 American households, it was found that 29 per cent of the diets did not furnish enough calcium; 10 per cent, not enough iron; 16 per cent, not enough vitamin A; 17 per cent, not enough vitamin B; and 25 per cent, not enough vitamin C.

Dr. Inez Eckblad of Washington State University found in her survey of teen-agers' diets that American youth's intake in terms of food values is only slightly better than those in the world's starvation areas. It is small wonder that the skin of American teen-agers is so loaded with blemishes.

Vitamin A

Vitamin A is a strong contributive factor in the prevention of premature aging, and therefore essential for a healthy skin. It aids the body in defense against infection, is necessary for normal liver function, and, along with C and E, gives protection against air pollution. Vitamin A brightens the whites of the eyes and keeps the eyes healthy. It protects the throat and lungs, and when deficient in vitamin A we constantly invite common colds because cells haven't the stamina to battle germs. Skin that is rough, with the appearance of "goose pimples," especially on the elbows, above the knees, buttocks, and upper arms is a sign of vitamin A deficiency. Also, dandruff and hair that is dry and brittle.

Foods highest in vitamin A are carrots, beet and dandelion greens, beef liver, calves' liver, spinach, tomatoes, sweet potatoes, green peppers, lettuce, winter squash, celery, cabbage, broccoli, alfalfa leaf meal, canteloupe, parsley, mustard greens, collards, endive, and fresh apricots.

Halibut liver oil has about a hundred times more vitamin A than cod liver oil. Both are sold with the number of units of vitamins A and D indicated on the label giving you a guideline for dosage. Keep any fish liver oil in the refrigerator to prevent its turning rancid.

The amount of vitamin A required by the human body has never been determined. In 1932 Mead Johnson offered a reward to anyone who could discover our requirement of vitamin A, and the offer was withdrawn twelve years later for lack of solution.

Improper absorption of vitamin A can be caused by infection, mineral oil, cold weather—and fat-free diets. As stated, vitamin A *needs* fat (found in vegetable oils) in order to dissolve. Anyone on a fat-free diet is inviting premature aging.

If you have any of the following, I suggest you consult a doctor in the practice of preventive medicine, or a nutritionist, regarding your intake of vitamin A . . . loss of pep, poor appetite, thyroid disorders, peeling or ridged nails, night blindness, excessive wrinkles, some types of hearing loss, and susceptibility to the common cold.

Many teen-age cases of acne have been cured by daily doses of brewers' yeast, vitamins A, B, C, and D, plus 300 mg. of pantothenic acid daily. Added to these have been zinc, plus a diet high in raw foods (fruits and vegetables), lean meat, fish, and fowl. And strict avoidance of fried foods. In the case of teen-age acne, it is imperative that the bowels remain open to prevent toxic accumulation in the intestines and colon. Such toxins can be reabsorbed into the system, starting the cycle all over again.

As a final note on vitamin A, research has indicated that it inhibits cancer, a discovery made when investigating environmental factors that cause cancer. Dr. Umberto Saffiotti, a pathologist at the Chicago Medical School, made the following report to the Ninth International Cancer Congress. Of 53 hamsters sprayed with a chemical found in industrial fumes, 16 developed lung cancer. But of 60 other hamsters given vitamin A following exposure to the carcinogens, 5 developed tumors, of which only 1 was malignant. There is also indication that vitamin A is effective in prevention of cancer of the cervix.

The B Vitamins

There is a complex of B vitamins; the basic ones are B_1, B_2, B_3, B_6 and B_{12}. *It is important to take the whole complex of B vitamins,* as they are necessary one to the other.

The B complex is water soluble and leaves the body on elimination. It is, therefore, vital that they be replaced—particularly if one is under physical or emotional stress. There isn't a better or easier way to do this than the daily intake of brewers' yeast. Rich in nucleic acids, brewers' yeast retards degenerative disease, recharges the cells, and gives optimum health as well as a beautiful skin.

I take two tablespoons of brewers' yeast every day, in a variety of ways. I mix it with any fresh citrus juice, and particularly enjoy it in a glass of tomato juice with a squeeze of lemon and dash of Tabasco. It's also good in a glass of raw milk with a bit of vanilla added. I supplement the brewers' yeast with RNA.

This daily habit was begun after I learned from Dr. Benjamin Frank's book, *Nucleic Acid Therapy in Aging and Degenerative Disease,* of the fantastic results obtained from his formula. My skin almost immediately looked smoother and rosier, and wrinkles diminished after two or three weeks. The skin over my whole body, including hands, showed remarkable improvement. His recommendation: B complex capsules taken daily at noon, plus RNA, 5–10 gr. taken twice weekly.

The B vitamins are rapidly depleted from the body by the intake of both alcohol and refined sugar. You might well be deficient in B vitamins if you are tired, nervous, depressed—or if you have acne or an exceptionally dry skin.

In addition to brewers' yeast, you can, of course, get B complex in pill form, and in certain foods—eggs, apples, cheese, watercress, carrots, grapefruit, fish, cabbage, whole grains, wheat germ and blackstrap molasses.

Here is a breakdown of the B vitamins.

B_1, KNOWN AS THIAMINE

B_1 converts carbohydrates into energy, is essential to reproductive power and nerve function, improves muscle tone and stamina, aids in proper elimination, and is a preventive of air and sea sickness. It has been called the "morale vitamin" because its lack results in depression, irritability, fatigue, and inability to concentrate. B_1 is found in whole grains, oatmeal, brown rice, egg yolks, wheat germ, and nuts (black walnuts, pecans, and hazel nuts). But brewers' yeast is the richest source. Without sufficient B_1, the body is not getting energy from sugar, and this results in a craving for sweets.

B_2, KNOWN AS RIBOFLAVIN

Like B_1, B_2 helps convert sugar and starches to energy. It aids in assimilation of iron and proteins and helps in the metabolism process. It is essential for healthy skin, hair and eyes. Lack of B_2 makes us more susceptible to infectious diseases. B_2 is found in wheat germ, peanuts, blueberries, dried prunes, cheese, eggs, apples, milk, whole grains, soy flour, hickory nuts, and the glandular parts of a steer. And, of course, brewers' yeast. B_2 is needed particularly by those suffering from oily skin and hair, dandruff, any burning sensation in the eyes when exposed to bright light, ulcers, and sores in corners of the mouth. The more fat in your diet, the greater your need for B_2. Here is a chart illustrating the amount of B_1 and B_2 available from sample foods. Notice the high content in brewers' yeast.

	B_1 per 100 grams	B_2 per 100 grams
Brewers' yeast	5,000 to 8,000	2,500 to 4,700
Lean pork	300 to 750	200
Dried lima beans	450 to 600	790
Liver	300 to 420	1,800 to 2,200

(Reprinted from *The Prevention Method for Better Health* c 1960 by J. I. Rodale. Permission granted by Rodale Press, Inc., Emmaus, Pa. 18049)

B_3, KNOWN AS NIACIN

B_3 is an aid in treating vertigo, increases circulation, can reduce cholesterol levels, and, as tested by a doctor in England, has cured acne. A deficiency of B_3 sometimes induces pellagra, once a widespread disease causing dermatitis, diarrhea, and psychic disturbances. When taken alone and without other B complex vitamins, however, large doses of B_3 are suspected as the cause of colitis and jaundice. I repeat, it is important to take B complex vitamins in balance, which is provided in all B complex capsules. The best sources of B_3 are brewers' yeast, veal, turkey, mushrooms, wheat bran, peanut butter, lamb, whole-wheat flour, mackerel, and swordfish. One of the functions of niacin is the formation of enzymes that are part of the chemical chain that assimilates sugars and starches. Therefore, the more sugar and starches you eat, the greater your need for B_3.

B_6, KNOWN AS PYRIDOXINE

B_6 regulates the production of histamines, which, in turn, regulate blood pressure, heart rate, and width of the arteries. B_6 is helpful in the cure of acne, helps prevent tooth decay, is an important source of energy. It aids the body to assimilate protein and helps fluid reduction. Therefore, it is a help for those attempting to lose weight. It is effective in relief of premenstrual tension. B_6 is found in liver, lima beans, bananas, brewers' yeast, wheat germ, sweet potatoes, peanuts, molasses. Deficiency of B_6 can cause a lot of woes. Among them, vaginal dermatitis, flatus, excessively oily skin, diabetes, and low blood pressure as well as muscular weakness. The Pill is often responsible for a deficiency in B_6.

B_{12}, KNOWN AS COBALAMIN

Discovered only recently (1948), B_{12} combats anemia. It is a vital supplement to the diet of strict vegetarians. Injections of B_{12} have been found to relieve and sometimes entirely clear bronchial asthma, hay fever, and rashes. It is found in meat, fish, chicken, turkey, dairy products, seeds, sprouts, and certain nuts—and it has recently been found that B_{12} is present in kelp in such quantity that two to three ounces of seaweed daily might be sufficient to provide the requirements of vegetarians.

Additional members of the B complex:

FOLIC ACID

Folic acid is necessary for the division of body cells, and for production of substances that carry RNA and DNA. It is found in green vegetables, particularly asparagus and dried limas. Also in canteloupe, liver, tortula, yeast, and nuts. It is destroyed by exposure to light and by heat (in cooking)—which is why it's important that we eat lots of raw foods—and by many drugs; phenobarbital and Dilantin among them.

PANTOTHENIC ACID

Pantothenic acid apparently occurs in all living cells—in yeasts, mold, bacteria, and individual cells of all plants and animals. It works in conjunction with B_2 and seems to alleviate problems of constipation because lack of it interferes with intestinal bacteria important in keeping a good balance in the intestinal tract. Like other B vitamins, it dissolves in water and is lost when water in which food has been cooked is drained away. Just as baking soda destroys all B vitamins, pantothenic acid is destroyed immediately when baking soda is added to food. Highest sources of pantothenic acid are egg yolks, liver, brewers' yeast, rice, bran, dried peas, Irish potatoes, wheat bran, whole fresh eggs, and cowpeas.

PABA (PARA-AMINOBENZOIC ACID)

PABA is an antagonist to sulfa drugs, and if it arrives first in the system and in greater quantity, the sulfa drug becomes ineffective. PABA helps intestinal bacteria to produce folic acid, which, in turn, helps the body to assimilate pantothenic acid. It becomes a chain reaction, and a chain is only as strong as its weakest link, so it is essential that all the B vitamins are in the body at all times in sufficient amount to be properly utilized. Foods high in PABA are liver, brewers' yeast, milk, eggs, rice bran, whole wheat, wheat germ, and molasses.

Vitamin C

Vitamin C helps the body use minerals and other vitamins for optimum nutrition. It is also important in the assimilation of medications. By itself, C is invaluable in aiding the system to detoxify from atmospheric poisons such as lead and mercury. Vitamin C maintains the health of bones, teeth, skin, tendons, blood vessel walls, cartilage, and collagen, and is perhaps most famous—since Dr. Pauling's pronouncement—for staving off colds and relieving their symptoms once they are incurred. Insofar as our appearance is concerned, and particularly the skin, C is invaluable because it is essential for the formation of collagen, which, as you've read, is the protein that holds us together. Without vitamin C, collagen does not function properly and skin sags, blotches, and is marred by broken capillaries. A deficiency of C is indicated by early morning bags beneath the eyes. Without C, cells and capillaries are fragile and fill with water. Without it, we are also subject to acne, dermatitis, psoriasis, and the pigment of the skin paling.

Each of us needs vitamin C in varying amounts, depending on metabolism and life style. But all of us need it to prevent premature aging of the skin. If I may include a personal pitch for C, I can tell you that after morning exercises I noticed small cutaneous hemorrhaging on my face, especially beneath the eyes. I increased my dosage of vitamin C and the small hemorrhages ceased—then showed up again when I made the test of returning to my previous dosage.

Vitamin C is found in rose hips, a plant obtainable at HFS in tea form. Foods containing vitamin C are citrus fruit, bell peppers, brussels sprouts, fresh grapefruit juice, mustard and dandelion greens, turnip tops, and almost all fresh vegetables in varying degrees.

A note of interest: If you take aspirin, it completely nullifies the effects of vitamin C. So if you have a cold, don't take aspirin if you are taking vitamin C.

Vitamin D

Vitamin D is necessary for calcification of the bones, which it does by regulating the absorption and metabolism of calcium and phosphorous, the bone-forming elements. It's, therefore, essential for correct tooth formation and bone growth, and it governs muscular action through its control of calcium content in the blood. It is necessary for proper glandular function, and essential for pregnant women.

The precise composition of vitamin D is unknown, but we do know we get D from rays of the sun. Ultraviolet rays transform subcutaneous fat into vitamin D. Too much vitamin D can be toxic; the daily intake should not exceed 5,000 International Units. However, most nutritionists agree that the recommended daily dosage of 400 IU is not sufficient. Without enough, the bones soften, there is lack of stamina, muscular weakness, instability of the nervous system, and muscle cramps.

A fat-soluble vitamin, D is stored in the liver. It is found in butter, milk, egg yolk, fish, meat, and fish liver oils. There is practically no vitamin D in most vegetables, cereals, and fruit. If you live in a climate with long and severe winters, I would recommend you take cod liver oil as a supplement for vitamin D.

D is needed by calcium; without D, calcium is not properly absorbed by the body. D should not be taken without its helpmate, vitamin A, so buy vitamin A and D together in a supplement.

Vitamin E

Vitamin E actually replaces moisture lost by the skin. If an E capsule is opened and its contents mixed with a moisturizer and then applied to the skin, it is an excellent conditioner. It has been found to heal skin ulcers and bedsores, and is very effective in healing burns. Both varicose veins and phlebitis have responded to 300–500 mg. of vitamin E daily. E has gained a reputation for arresting the aging process: research demonstrates that it prevents oxygen from forming toxic compounds, which interfere with cell respiration. The greatest percentage of E is concentrated in the adrenal glands, which regulate sodium and potassium, help the body respond to stress, and produce sex hormones.

Vitamin E is found in wheat germ, whole grains, eggs, brown rice, salad greens, and the oils of corn, peanuts, soybeans, and cottonseed.

An oil-soluble vitamin, E can be destroyed in fried fats and fried oils in the diet. It is also destroyed by bleaching agents used in white flour, by sulfa drugs, and by mineral oil. If you take a supplement with iron, take vitamin E twelve hours before or after the iron intake, as the type of iron given for anemia demolishes vitamin E.

Lack of E can cause sterility and coronary disease. And it should be noted that E (as well as the B vitamins) works more efficiently when the body has a sufficient supply of vitamin C.

Vitamin F

We could not exist without vitamin F. It combines with proteins and cholesterol to form structures so basic that there is no life without them. One of these is the membrane that encloses every living cell. If such a membrane is absent, weak, or faulty, the cell dies. Vitamin F forms myelin, a fatty protein substance that sheaths the major nerves, including the spinal cord. Healthy nerves cannot exist without vitamin F. It is found in milk, butter, beef fat, wheat germ, and all oils, such as linseed, corn, coconut, peanut, olive, etc.

Vitamin K

Vitamin K is the vitamin necessary for proper coagulation of the blood. Certain antibiotics, which interfere or can destroy beneficial intestinal flora, have made the manufacture of vitamin K in the body less reliable than it was prior to the introduction of antibiotics. Our systems can manufacture their own vitamin K, but we need healthy intestinal flora for this.

Foods high in vitamin K are spinach, kale, alfalfa, cabbage, cauliflower, green peas, carrot tops, liver, eggs, soybean oil, and blackstrap molasses.

Vitamin P

Vitamin P is a substance occurring along with vitamin C in foods. It is most commonly known as the bioflavonoids. These are the brightly colored substances in fruits—are also found in the white portion of the orange and grapefruit, etc. It's better to eat an orange than to drink its juice. Bioflavonoids are important to the health of the capillaries.

Rutin is another part of vitamin P. It, too, is necessary for health of capillaries, and has been shown to help hypertension. It is also essential in treatment of hemorrhaging due to disease. Rutin keeps company with vitamin C; it is found wherever nature has supplied vitamin C. Foods high in P are fruits, particularly prunes, black and white grapes, black currants, and citrus fruits. Vitamin P is also found in rose hips.

MINERALS

Although the body can manufacture some of the vitamins, it is unable to produce its own minerals, which must be supplied by diet. Minerals are sometimes called "trace elements" because they are present in such minute quantities . . . mostly in bones, teeth, and cartilage. They are important in the overall functioning and acid/alkaline balance of the body.

Our supply of minerals is higher while we are young, and the cells are replaced as rapidly as they die. With increasing age, our mineral supply diminishes and cell growth slows. Wrinkles form when dead cells are not replaced; ergo, minerals can be considered one of the keys to youthfulness.

If one of these elements is missing, the entire balance can be disrupted, causing problems with skin among other organs. It is necessary to take a supplement of both vitamins and minerals in proper ratio. Any physician who is nutritionally oriented can steer you to selection of such a supplement.

"In the absence of minerals," says Charles Northen, M.D., "vitamins have no function. Lacking vitamins, the system can make use of minerals—but lacking minerals, the vitamins are useless." We have only a few ounces of vitamins in our system but almost six pounds of minerals. So you can see how important minerals are. They are truly the key to a more youthful you.

Calcium

Calcium must have vitamins A, C, D, and phosphorous in the proper ratio, which is twice as much calcium as phosphorous. (There is more calcium in our bodies than any other mineral.)

Phosphorous

Phosphorous is present in every body cell, working to neutralize excess blood acidity and metabolizing fats and starches. Refined sugar is lethal to both calcium and phosphorous because it destroys the ratio.

Sodium

Without sodium, which helps the manufacture of hydrochloric acid, carbohydrate foods cannot be changed into fat for the digestive process. Along with potassium, sodium helps keep a correct fluid balance in the body.

Potassium

Potassium works with sodium in keeping proper fluid balance. Most diuretics destroy potassium, and lack of this essential mineral can upset the entire nervous system.

Magnesium

Magnesium plays an important part, as a co-enzyme, in building protein. Many mental and emotional disorders are improved with the intake of magnesium. Alcoholism is also treated with magnesium diet because alcohol destroys magnesium. Foods rich in magnesium are nuts, seeds, apples, celery, figs, grapefruit, and yellow corn.

Iron

Iron is necessary for the correct functioning of blood. If skin is too pale or sallow, this might indicate a dearth of iron. In order to function, iron must have sufficient calcium.

Richest sources of iron are liver, wheat germ, food yeast, eggs, and turnip greens.

Iodine

Iodine is vital for proper stimulation of the thyroid gland, enabling it to secrete thyroxine, the hormone that regulates metabolism and energy. Deficiency of iodine can cause goiter, obesity, and sluggish metabolism.

Fish, shellfish, sea water, kelp, and seaweed are rich in iodine:

Copper

Once iron has helped in the creation of blood, it is copper that is needed to convert the blood into hemoglobin. Without copper, vitamin C would not be properly assimilated.

Sources of copper are egg yolks, dried peas and beans, whole wheat, prunes, and almonds.

Manganese

Manganese works with the B vitamins to give energy and is necessary to the job of the enzymes so that food can be well digested and utilized by the body. A deficiency of manganese causes defect in the function of the pancreas.

Foods rich in manganese are brewers' yeast, dried peas and beans, egg yolks, green-leafed vegetables, and unmilled grains.

Zinc

A metallic element, zinc is a micronutrient and a powerful catalyst, directing the efficiency of body processes and the maintenance of enzymes. It is an antitoxin for some types of drug poisoning, including marijuana and hashish. Zinc is concentrated within the thyroid gland, but amounts of it are also in the hair, skin, blood, and nervous system.

Much zinc is destroyed in food processing—over 80 per cent loss in white bread. Chemical fertilizers used in agriculture prevent plants from absorbing zinc. Some farmers add zinc to the feed of their livestock—we have to furnish it for ourselves.

Appendix

GUIDE TO MEAL PLANNING

(*See following lists for protein foods, vegetables A and B, cereals, and fruits allowed*)

Before breakfast, a glass of pure water at room temperature.

	1,000 Calories	1,200 Calories	1,500 Calories
BREAKFAST			
Citrus juice or, preferably, apple juice			
or	1 serving	1 serving	1 serving
1 piece of fruit	1 serving	1 serving	1 serving
or			
Protein food	1 serving	1 serving	1 serving
Whole-grain wheat toast, 1 slice	1 serving	1 serving	1 serving
or			
Cereal	1 serving	1 serving	1 serving
Butter or oil	None	½ serving	1 serving
LUNCH			
Protein food	1 serving	1 serving	1 serving
Vegetable (*list B*)	1 serving	1 serving	1 serving
or			
Whole-grain bread, 1 slice	1 serving	1 serving	1 serving
1 piece of fruit	1 serving	2 servings	2 servings
Butter or oil	1 serving	1 serving	3 servings
Skim milk or buttermilk	1 cup	1 cup	1 cup

DINNER

Fasting broth *	1 cup	1 cup	1 cup
Protein food	2 servings	2 servings	2 servings
Vegetable (*list A*)	As desired	As desired	As desired
Vegetable (*list B*)	1 serving	1 serving	1 serving
Bread or carbohydrate	1 serving	1 serving	1 serving
Fruit	(if none at lunch) 1 serving	(if none at lunch) 1 serving	(if none at lunch) 1 serving
Butter or oil	None	1½ servings	2 servings
Skim milk or buttermilk	1 cup	1 cup	1 cup

Vegetables—A list

(*Any amount if raw—if cooked, ½ to 1 cup daily*)

	Calories
Artichokes, 4 hearts	20
Asparagus, canned—1 cup	43
Asparagus, fresh—1 cup	36
Beans, green, canned—1 cup	27
Beans, green, fresh—1 cup	27
Bean sprouts—½ cup	15
Broccoli—1 cup	33
Brussels sprouts—1 cup	44
Burdock root—3½ oz.	94
Cabbage (celery or Chinese) cooked—1 cup	27
Cabbage (celery or Chinese) raw	14
Cauliflower—1 cup	30
Celery—1 cup	18
Chard, cooked—1 cup	30
Cucumber—1 medium	18
Dandelion greens—1 cup	79
Eggplant—3½ oz.	24

* See page 6 for recipe.

	Calories
Garlic—1 clove	5
Lettuce—2 large leaves	6.8
Mung bean sprouts—4 oz.	10
Mushrooms—1 cup	20
Okra—1 cup	32
Peppers, green—1 whole	16
Radishes—4 small	4
Sauerkraut—1 cup	32
Summer squash—1 cup	22
Tomato—1 small	22
Zucchini—½ cup	23

Vegetables—B list

(½ cup daily)

	Calories
Beets, canned—1 cup	68
Beets, fresh—1 cup	58
Carrots—1 cup	45
Corn—1 ear fresh	84
Corn—½ cup canned	70
Onions—1 tbs. raw	4
1 Bermuda, raw	49
1 Spanish	8
6 small green	23
Parsnips—1 cup	94
Peas, fresh—3½–4 oz.	98
Rutabagas	50
Squash, winter—1 cup	60
Turnips—1 cup	42

Fruits allowed

	Calories
Apples—1 small	60
Applesauce, unsweetened—½ cup	50

	Calories
Apricots, fresh—3 medium	54
Bananas—1 medium	88
Berries (most)—1 cup	83
Cantaloupe—½ medium	37
Cherries—1 cup	65
Dates—2	65
Figs, fresh—3 large	100
Grapefruit—½ small	104
Grapes, Concord—1 cup	84
Mango—1 medium	87
Melons, Casaba— 2″ x 7″ wedge	52
Honeydew— 2″ x 7″ wedge	49
Persian— 2″ x 7″ wedge	52
Musk— 2″ x 7″ wedge	37
Nectarine—1 medium	38
Orange—1 large	106
Papaya—1 cup	71
Peach—1 medium	46
Pear—1 small	96
Pineapple—1 cup	74
Plum—1 cup	94
Prunes—2	36
Tangerines—1 medium	35
Watermelon—½ slice, 1″ thick	45
Cereals—4 oz.	

Cereals and Breads

All-Bran—4 oz.	73
Bran Flakes, 40% bran	57

	Calories
Raisin Bran	75
Bran, whole cereal, cooked	113
Grapenuts	200
Oatmeal, cooked	74
Ralston Health	100
Roman Meal	135
Scotch oatmeal, cooked	150
Wheatgerm—¼ cup	63
Wheatena, cooked—1 cup	120

Breads—one slice

	Calories
Bran	53
Rye	57
Soya	65
Swedish Health	51
Mexican tortilla	50

Juices

(3½ oz.)

	Calories	Vitamin & Mineral Content
Apple	47	Potassium
Apricot	57	Potassium, vitamin A
Beet	26	Potassium, sodium
Beet tops	24	Potassium, sodium, calcium, vitamin A
Blackberry	37	Potassium
Cabbage	24	Potassium, vitamin A
Carrot	42	Potassium, vitamin A
Celery	17	Potassium, sodium, vitamin A

	Calories	Vitamin & Mineral Content
Cherry	58	Potassium, vitamin A
Coconut	22	Potassium, sodium,
Cranberry	46	Potassium, sodium, vitamin A
Grape	183	Potassium, calcium, phosphorous
Grapefruit	39	Potassium, vitamins A, C
Lemon	25	Potassium, phosphorous, vitamins A, C
Orange	45	Potassium, sodium, calcium, phosphorous, vitamins A, C
Papaya	39	Potassium, calcium, phosphorous, sodium vitamins A, C
Parsley (HFS)	44	Potassium, calcium, phosphorous, sodium, iron, vitamins A, C
Pear (nectar)	52	Potassium, calcium, phosphorous, vitamin A
Pineapple	55	Potassium, calcium, phosphorous, vitamins A, C
Prune	77	Potassium, calcium, phosphorous, sodium, iron, vitamin C
Tangerine	43	Potassium, calcium, phosphorous, sodium, vitamin C
Tomato	19	Potassium, calcium, phosphorous, sodium, vitamins A, C

(*Note by JV* Calories as well as mineral content differ, depending on type of vegetable or fruit, when harvested, and soil grown in. These were computed as close as possible. In all instances, the raw calorie value was taken as there was no data on juice.)

APPENDIX

Protein Food

	Calories	Grams of Protein in 3½ oz.
Cottage cheese,		
creamed—½ cup	115	13.6
skimmed—½ cup	86	17.0
Cheese, blue or roquefort	368	21.5
brick	370	22
Swiss	355	26.4
parmesan	393	36
Brewers' yeast—1 tbs.	22	8
Yoghurt, plain		
partially skim milk	50	3.4
partially whole milk	63	3.0
Milk—4 oz.		
Whole	65	3.5
Acidophilus	100	3.5
Skim	36	3.6
Buttermilk	36	3.6
Cream (half and half)—2 tbs.	48	1.1
Eggs		
Poached—2 medium	163	12.7
Hard boiled—2 medium	163	12.7
Scrambled	173	11.2
Raw	163	12.9
Seafood (boiled, broiled, steamed, or raw)		
Abalone—3½ oz.	107	18.7
Anchovies, 6 small	65	5.7
Bass, striped	196	21.5
Bass, black sea	259	15.8
Bluefish	159	26.2

	Calories	Grams of Protein in 3½ oz.
Catfish	103	17.6
Clams, canned and drained	98	15.8
Cod	170	28.5
Crab, canned	101	17.4
Crab (blue, Dungeness, rock, king)	93	17.3
Flatfish (sole, flounder, sand dabs)	79	16.7
Flounder	202	30.0
Frog legs	73	16.4
Haddock	165	19.6
Halibut	171	25.2
Lobster	194	18.5
Mackerel, broiled, 1 tbs. butter	236	21.8
Mussels, canned, drained	114	18.2
Oysters, canned, solids and liquid	76	8.5
Perch, white	91	18.5
Pike	90	19.1
Red snapper	93	19.5
Salmon	222	19.1
Scallops	112	23.2
Shad	201	23.2
Shrimp—3½ oz.	91	18.1
Sturgeon, smoked	149	31.2
Swordfish	174	28.0
Tuna, canned, in oil	197	28.8
Tuna, canned, in water	127	28.0
Whitefish	215	15.2

	Calories	Grams of Protein in 3½ oz.
Fowl (roasted)		
Chicken, without skin,		
Light meat	166	31.6
Dark meat	176	28.0
Turkey, light meat	176	32.9
Turkey, dark meat	203	30.0
Meat (roasted, broiled, or pan fried)		
Hamburger	219	27.4
Porterhouse steak	465	19.7
T-bone steak	473	19.5
Club steak	454	20.6
Flank steak	196	30.5
Round steak	261	28.6
Rump	347	23.6
Lamb, leg	319	23.2
Lamb chop	492	16.9
Veal loin chop	234	26.4
Veal rib chop	269	27.2

ON FOOD COMBINATIONS

1. Do not eat proteins with starch.
2. Do not eat fruit and vegetables at the same meal. Different enzymes are used in digestion, possibly causing flatulence.
3. Milk combines poorly with anything and should be consumed separately.
4. Do not mix sweet fruits (figs, bananas, dates) with acid fruits (citrus). Eat each group separately.
5. Starches and sugars may be combined with vegetables.
6. Fruit should be eaten alone, except for combining it with nuts.

Foods	Combine Best With	Combine Poorly With
Meat, all kinds	Green vegetables	Milk, starches, sweets, other proteins, acid fruits, acid vegetables butter, cream, oils
Nuts	Green vegetables, acid fruits	Milk, starches, sweets, other proteins, acid foods, butter, cream, oils
Eggs	Green vegetables	Milk, starches, sweets, other proteins, acid foods, butter, cream, oils
Cheese	Green vegetables	Starches, sweets, other proteins, acid foods, butter, cream, oils
Milk, best taken alone	Fair with fruits	All proteins, starches, vegetables
Cereals, all kinds, are best eaten alone		All foods
Fats, oils, butter, cream	All starches, vegetables	All proteins
Legumes, beans (except green beans) peas	Green vegetables	All proteins, sweets, milk fruits, butter, cream, oils
Melons, all kinds	The one fruit that should be eaten alone	
Fruits, sweet	Milk, sweet or sour	Acid fruits, starches, cereals, bread, potatoes, proteins
Fruits, acid	Other acid fruits, fair with nuts, milk	Sweets, starches, cereals, bread, potatoes, all proteins except nuts
Green vegetables	All proteins, all starches	Milk, fruit
Starches	Green vegetables, fats, oils	Proteins, fruits, acids, sugars

FOOD CLASSIFICATIONS

Carbohydrates

Carbohydrates are the starches and sugars. They are broken up into three groups: (1) starches, (2) sugars and syrups, and (3) sweet fruits.

STARCHY
All cereals, dry beans (except soy beans), dry peas, potatoes, chestnuts, peanuts, peanuts, pumpkins, hubbard squash, banana squash, Jerusalem artichokes.

MILDLY STARCHY
Cauliflower, beets, carrots, rutabaga

SUGARS AND SYRUPS
Brown sugar, milk sugar, white sugar (an untouchable), honey, maple syrup, cane syrup.

SWEET FRUITS
Bananas, dates, figs, raisins, grapes (Thompson and Muscat), prunes, sun-dried pears, persimmons.

Fats

Safflower oil, olive oil, soy oil, sunflower seed oil, corn oil, avocadoes, lard, nut oils, butter, cottenseed oil, fat meats, pecans and most nuts.

Acid Fruits

Most of the acid eaten as food comes from the acid fruits. Orange, grapefruit, pineapple, pomegranate, tomato, lemon, lime, sour apple, sour grape, sour peach, sour plum.

Sub-acid Fruits

Fig, pear, cherry, papaya, sweet peaches, sweet apples, apricots, sweet plum, huckleberry, mango.

Non-starchy and Green Vegetables
All succulent vegetables, without regard to color, are in this classification. Lettuce, celery, endive, chicory, cabbage, cauliflower, broccoli, Brussels sprouts, collards, spinach, dandelion, beet tops, turnip tops, kohlrabi, sweet pepper, okra, cowslip, chinese cabbage, chive, mustard, leeks, turnips, kale, mullein, green corn, eggplant, green beans, cucumbers, radishes, sorrel, parsley, rhubarb, onions, watercress, scallions, garlic, zucchini, escarole, bamboo sprouts, summer squash, chard.

Index

A, vitamin, 9, 179, 180–81, 188; deficiency symptoms, 180–81; need for and food sources of, 180–81
Acid fruits, 201; sub-acid, 201
Acne, 64–66; causes, 64; mash #1, 65; mash #2, 65; treatment, 64–65, vitamins and, 65, 181
Agar-agar, 76, 169
Aging. See Longevity
Air pollution, skin care and, 47
Alcohol (alcoholism), 7–8
Aloe vera plant, 54, 169–70
Amino acids, 8; for hair, 75
Ankles, exercise for, 145
Answer—Preventive Medicine, The (Cleave, Campbell, and Painters), 38
Arm and leg raises, 28
Arms (arm muscles, corrective exercises for, 135, 138
Aspirin, avoiding use of, 45; vitamin C and, 185
Athlete's foot, 162
Aveeno, 55, 170

B (B complex), vitamins, 8, 9, 179–80, 181–85; B_1 (thiamine), 181, 182, 183; B_2 (riboflavin), 181, 182, 183; B_3 (niacin), 183; B_6 (pyridoxine), 8, 44, 181, 183; B_{12} (cobalamin), 181, 184; defi-

B (B complex (Continued)
ciencies, 182; folic acid, 9, 184; need for and food sources of, 181–85; paba, 58, 80, 184–85; pantothenic acid, 76, 161, 184
Bags under the eyes, 90. See also Wrinkles
Baking soda douche, 156
Baldness, 79
Basil, 170
Bathing, cleanliness and, 6–7, 153–55. See also Cleanliness; Showers
Bathing suits, 148
Baths, cool, sunburn and, 53, 55
Beer shampoo, 75
Bioflavinoids, 187
Birth control pill. See Pill, the
Black, Karen, 93
Black eyes (shiners), 91
Blackheads, 64
Bleach(ing): eyebrows, 94–95; hair (see under Hair)
Blond hair: lightener, 82; toner, 82
Blood circulation, exercises for, 12, 25
Blood pressure, high. See High blood pressure
Body makeup, removing, 158
Body odor (see also Perspiration): deodorants for, 155–56
Bone meal, 42

Bone structure (body build). *See* Figure
Bras, clothes and figure and, 148, 150
Breads and cereals, meal-planning guide and calories and, 194–95
Breasts. *See* Bust
Brewers' yeast, use of, 41, 42, 43, 49, 161, 181, 183, 184, 189, 197
Broth, fasting, 6
Brushing (brushes): hair, 71, 72, 73, 74; makeup, 98; massage and, 154
Bubble baths, 154
Burdock root, 170; tea, 65
Burkitt, Dr. Denis, 127
Bust: bras and, 148, 150; clothes and, 148; exercises for, 136–39; plastic surgery and, 149–51; posture and, 145–46
Buttocks. *See* Hips; Thighs

C, vitamin, 3, 179–80, 181, 185, 186, 187, 188; need for and food sources of, 8, 9, 185, 196
Calcium, 9, 43, 65, 127, 186, 188; lactate, 9, 161; need for and food sources of, 161, 188, 195, 196
Calluses, 162
Calories: meal-planning guide and, 191–99; weight and (*see* Overweight)
Calves, exercise for, 145
Cameras. *See* Photography
Camomile, 170; tea, 170
Cancer: diet and, 127; hair dyes and, 81; red clover and, 171; skin, 46; vitamin A and, 181
Carbohydrates, 37–38, 40, 179, 201 (*see also* specific kinds); refined and natural, 37–38; starches and sugars, 38, 40, 201
Carne, Judy, 1
Carrots, 90, 193
Castor oil, for eyebrows, 95
Celandine, 91, 170–71
Cereals and breads, meal-planning guide and calories and, 194–95
Cheese, 197, 200
Chelated vitamins and minerals, 8, 9
Chelation process, 171
Cher, 4, 86, 150
Chicken. *See* Fowl
Chin: double (*see* Double chin); makeup for problem areas, 108–9, 124
Chlorine, swimming and hair care and, 80

Chlorophyl, 156, 174
Cholesterol, 126, 171; lecithin and, 171, 173
Cider vinegar, for sunburn, 54
"City skin," 47
Cleanliness, 153–58; bathing and, 6–7, 153–55; clothes, 158; deodorants, 155–56; Epsom salt bath, 155; feet, 154, 162–64; fingernails, 161; fragrance, 153, 157; hair, 71–72, 73–75, 85; hands, 160; herbal baths and, 153–54, 155; oil bath, 155; shaving and, 156–57; skin, 47–52ff.; teeth, 157–58
Cleansers, skin, 47–48; acne, 65; dry skin, 48; oily skin, 48
Cleave, Campbell, and Painters, 38
Clothes (wardrobe), 147–49; cleanliness and, 158; photography and, 124
Clover, 171; red, 171; white, 171
Cobalamin. *See under* B (B complex) vitamins
"Cobra, the," 26–27
Cod liver oil, 180, 186
Colbert, Claudette, 83
Colds, 74; vitamins and, 181, 185
Collagen, 7, 49, 90, 185
Colman, Ronald, 159
Color (coloring), hair, 80–82
Color chart, makeup, 104–5
Colostomy, 40
Combs (combing), hair care and, 72, 74. *See also* Brushing
Comfrey, 154, 171
Conditioners, hair, henna as, 81
Contact lenses, 92, 93
Copper, dietary, 189
Corn meal, for dry shampoo, 75
Corns and calluses, 162
Coronary disease. *See* Heart problems
Corrective exercises. *See* Exercises; specific body areas, exercises, problems
Cosmetics, 98 (*see also* Makeup); color chart, 104–5
Cosmetic surgery. *See* Plastic surgery
Crane, Hart, 89
Crawford, Joan, 94
Crepe neck, exercise for, 57
Cucumber slices, for eyes, 91
Curlers, hair, 87
Cuts (cutting), hair, 85–87

D, vitamin, 9, 181, 185–86, 188; need for and food sources of, 185–86
Dairy products, 39 (see also specific kinds); calories and protein in (listed), 197
Dandruff: egg shampoo for, 75; herbs for, 174, 175, 176
Deneuve, Catherine, 1
Deodorants, use of, 155–56
Depilatory, use of, 156–57
Dermatitis urbis ("city skin"), 47
Detergents. See Soaps
Dewhurst, Colleen, 84
Diaphragm breathing, 167
Diction. See Voice
Diet (food). See Food
Dieting (diets), 125–26 (see also Food; Overweight); fasting and, 6–8; meal-planning guide and, 191
Digestive system (see also Elimination): fasting and, 6
Diverticulosis, 40
DNA. See RNA and DNA
Double chin: exercise for, 57, 58; makeup for, 109, 124
Douche, 156
Dress (clothes, wardrobe), 147–49. See also Clothes
Drinking. See Alcohol (alcoholism)
Drinks (beverages, liquids, juices): fruit juices (see Fruit and fruit juices); meal-planning guide and calories and, 195–96; milk (see Milk); skin shake, 49, 161; vegetable (see under Vegetables); water, 6, 8, 9
Drugs, avoiding use of, 3, 44–45
Dryers, hair, 74
Dry hair: egg shampoo for, 75; herbal rinse for, 78
Dry shampoo, 75
Dry skin: cleansers, 48; facials, 51–52
Duke, Patty, 3
Duncan, Sandy, 3
Dyes, hair, 80–82

E, vitamin, 8, 9, 186; need for and food sources of, 186
Ear wiggling exercise, 61
Eating habits. See Food
Eckblad, Dr. Inez, 180
Eczema, herbs for, 170, 173

Egg(s), 39, 179, 197, 200; in diet, 39, 179, 197, 200; in facials, 51–52; shampoo, 75
Elderflower, 172
Elimination: drinking water and, 8; fasting and, 6–7, 8
Energy, nutrition and, 37, 41
Enunciation. See Voice
Epsom salt bath, 155
Exercises, 9–35, 127–45 (see also specific body areas, kinds, problems); corrective, 128–45; eye, 91–92; face, 55–63; figure and weight and, 127–45; foot, 145, 163; stretch and pull, 11–14
Eyebright (herb), 91, 172
Eyebrows, 94–95; bleaching, 94–95; color, 94–95; locating orbital bone, 118; makeup, 99, 115, 118–20; penciling, 95; plucking (tweezing), 94, 118, 119, 120, 121
Eyelashes, makeup and, 103, 116, 117; curling, 103; mascara, 103, 116, 117
Eyelids, makeup and, 99, 101, 104–5, 115, 117; base for, 99; color chart, 104; curling lashes, 103; mascara, 103
Eyeliner, use of, 100, 116
Eyes (eye care), 89–95; bags and wrinkles, 90 (see also Wrinkles); black eyes (shiners), 91; contact lenses and eyeglasses, 92–93; exercises for, 91–92; fasting and, 90; foreign objects in, 90; glaucoma and, 89–90; herbal lotions and herbs for, 91, 172; makeup and, 98, 99, 115–17, 118, 119 (see also Eyebrows; Eyelashes; Eyelids); makeup color chart for, 104–5; night blindness and, 90; plastic surgery and, 93–94; problem areas, makeup for, 115–20; puffiness in, 90, 91; sunlight and, 92; tired, 91; vitamins and, 90
Eyeshadow, use of, 101–2; color chart for, 104

F, vitamin, 187
Fabray, Nanette, 68
Face (see also Chin; Eyes; Jaw; Lips; Mouth; Neck; Skin; Voice): acne and, 64–66; cleanliness and, 47–48; cleansers and fresheners, 47–48, 65; exercises, 55–62; facials, 48, 49–50 (see also Facials); hair style and shape of, 83; keeping hands away from, 159, 161;

Face (*Continued*)
lifts and peels, 67–69; makeup, 97–124 (*see also* Makeup); makeup color chart, 104–5; makeup for photography, 123–24; narrow, makeup for, 110; perspiration problem, 123; plastic surgery for, 66–69; problem areas, makeup for, 106–20; round, makeup for, 111; scrub, 48; wrinkles, 47 (*see also* Wrinkles)

Facials (facial masks), 48, 49–52; dry skin, 51; dry to normal skin, 51; formula for dry and scaly skin, 52; formula for dry skin, 51–52; fuller's earth, 50–51; oily skin, 52; rejuvenating, 50; sunburn, 54; tightener, 50

Farrow, Mia, 85

Fast food, 5

Fasting, 6–8, 37, 125; broth, 6; eyes and, 90; showering (cleanliness) and, 6–7, 15; vitamins and minerals and, 8–9; and weight loss, 7

Fats, body (blood), 38

Fats (oils), dietary, 179, 201; use on hair, 72

Fawcett, Farrah, 71, 86

Feet (foot care), 162–64; arches, 163; athlete's foot, 162; bath, 162; calluses and corns, 162; exercises, 145, 163; massage for, 163; pumice and hindu stones for, 162; soak, 162; tired, 162, 163; toenails, 163–64; and toxins, 154, 162

Fiber (bulk, roughage), dietary, 38, 40

Fields, Totie, 68

Figure (body build, bone structure), 125–51; clothes and, 147–49 (*see also* Clothes); corrective exercises for, 127–45 (*see also* Exercises); food and liquid intake and, 125–27, 145; plastic surgery and, 149–51 (*see also* Plastic surgery); posture and, 145–47; weight and, 125–27, 145 (*see also* Overweight)

Fingernails, 161; cream for, 161; filing, manicuring, 161; polish, 161; thin, calcium and gelatin for, 161

Finishing rinses, hair care and shampooing and, 74, 76–78; for falling hair, 79; herbal, 77–78; herbal for dry hair, 78; herbal for oily hair, 78; herbal ingredients, 76–77; rosemary, 77

Fish (*see also* Seafood): liver oils, 180, 186

Flour, refined, 37, 38

Folic acid, 9, 184

Food (diet, eating habits, nutrition), 5, 37–43 (*see also* specific aspects, classifications, kinds); classifications, 201–2; combinations, 40–41, 199–200; and dieting, 125–26, 191 (*see also* Dieting); and energy, 37, 41; and exercise, 145; fasting and (*see* Fasting); and figure, 125–27; and fingernails, 161; meal-planning guide and calories and, 191–99; and skin beauty and care, 37ff.; vitamins and minerals and (*see* Minerals: Vitamins; specific kinds, uses); and weight problem, 125–27, 145 (*see also* Overweight)

Foundation, makeup: applying, 99, 104; color chart, 104

Fowl (chicken, turkey), 39, 43; calories and protein in, 199

Fragrance (perfumes), 153, 157

Frank, Dr. Benjamin, 44

Freckles, papaya juice for, 175

Frown lines, 55, 56. *See also* Wrinkles

Fruit and fruit juices, 5, 40, 41, 42, 43, 201; acid and sub-acid, 201; combinations, 199, 200; meal-planning guide and calories and, 193–94, 195–96; sweet, 201

Fuller's earth, facial mask with, 50–51

Galsworthy, John, 89

Garbo, Greta, 166

Genital odor, 156

Glasses (eyeglasses), 92–93

Glaucoma, 89–90

Gleason, Jackie, 68

Glose, in agar-agar, 169

Golden seal (Hydrastis), 172

"Goose pimples," vitamin A and, 180

Gordon, Ruth, 84

Gray hair, coloring and, 80–82

Hair (and scalp), 71–87; blond toner, 82; brushing, 71, 72, 73; color (coloring), 80–82; conditioners, 73; cuts, 85–87; eyebrow, 94–95, 122 (*see also* Eyebrows); herbs for, 170–77 *passim;* lightener, 82; long or short, 84–85; loss of hair, 79; massage, 72, 74; mayonnaise for, 73; oil treatment, 72–73; oily and dry, 72, 73, 75; in photography,

INDEX

Hair (and scalp) *(Continued)*
83; pre-shampoo, 72–73; protein and, 71, 75; rinses for *(see* Finishing rinses); scalp massage and, 72, 74; setting, 87; shampooing and, 71–72, 73–75 *(see also* Shampooing); shaving, 156–57; style, 83–87; sunlight and, 80; wigs, 82–83
Hands (hand care), 159–60; cleaning, 160; fingernails, 161; handshake, 160; keeping away from the face, 159, 161; nourishing treatment for, 160
Head stand, 62
Heart problems (coronary disease, heart attacks): cholesterol and, 126; diet and, 38–39, 126; Rinse's formula for a healthy heart and, 41–42
Henna, 81, 172; neutral, 81; red, 81
Herbal baths, 153–54, 155
Herbal hair rinses, 76–78, 81–82; dry hair and, 78; falling hair and, 79; oily hair and, 78
Herbs (herbal teas), 41, 169–78 *(see also* Herbal baths; Herbal hair rinses; specific kinds, problems, uses); sources for ingredients, 177–78; what they are (listed), 169–77
High blood pressure (hypertension), vitamin E and, 9
Hips *(see also* Thighs): clothes and, 149; corrective exercises for, 140–42; exercises for, 19–20, 30–35, 140–42; plastic surgery and, 151
Histamines, vitamin B_6 and, 183
Honey, 38, 41; in hand-nourishing formula, 160
Horizontal scissors (exercise), 32–33
Hose, support, 163
Hunzas, the, 125
Hydrastis. *See* Golden seal
Hyssop bath, 153

Implants, breast, 150–51
Iodine, dietary, need for, 179, 189
Ions, negative and positive, bathing and, 154
Iron, dietary, need for, 189

Jaw, wide, makeup for, 109
Jogging, 10; in place, 10
Juices, fruit and vegetable *(see also* Fruit and fruit juices; Vegetables):

Juices *(Continued)*
meal-planning guide and calories and, 195–96

Kefir, 43, 172–73. *See also* Yoghurt
Kelp, 184
Keratin protein, for hair, 75
Khus khus, 173
Knee bends, 19–20; for thigh bulge, 143

Language, use of. *See* Voice
Lanolin, 98, 173
Lavender flowers, 154, 173
Laxatives, fasting and use of, 6
Leachman, Cloris, 3, 97
Lecithin, 42, 173; cholesterol and, 171, 173
Leg and arm raises, 28
Leg raises, 23–24, 145
Legs (leg problems): exercises for, 23–24, 28, 30–35, 145; hose for, 163; shaving, 156–57
Leg swing, 34–35
Lemon, 173; for corns and calluses, 162
Lemon grass, 174
Lenclos, Ninon de, herbal bath formula of, 154
Lifts, facial. *See under* Face
Linseed oil, natural, 79, 95
Lips, makeup for, 103, 112–14; brush, use of, 98; full, lipstick for, 113; irregular, lipstick for, 114; lipstick and gloss tones, color chart, 105; thin, lipstick for, 112
Liquid protein: diet, avoiding, 126; for hair, 71, 75
Liver, vitamins and, 180, 183
Longevity: food intake and weight and, 125–27; vitamins and, 180–81, 186
Loofa sponge, 6–7, 15, 154, 174
Loren, Sophia, 1, 95
Loss of hair, 79; rinse for falling hair, 79
Louise, Tina, 74

Magnesium, 127, 189
Makeup, 97–124; base, 99; body, removing, 158; brushes, 98; color chart, 104–5; cosmetics, 98; curling lashes, 103; equipment for, 98; eyeliner, 100, 116; eye pencil, 98, 99, 115; eyeshadow, 101–2, 104; fifteen-minute, 99–103; foundation, applying, 99, 104; lipstick,

Makeup (*Continued*)
103; mascara, 103, 116, 117; perspiration on face and, 123; photography and, 123–24; powder, 99, 103; problem areas and, 106–17; rouges, 99, 104; rule for, 97–98
Mammoplasty, 150–51
Manganese, 189
Manicure, 161
Mascara, use of, 103, 116, 117
Mask. *See* Facials
Massage, 154; foot, 163; scalp, 72, 74
Mastectomies, 151
Mayonnaise, as a hair conditioner, 73
Meat (meat eating), 39–40, 200; calories and protein in (listed), 199
Melons, 40–41, 200
Milk, 39, 197, 199, 200; effect on teeth of, 158
Mineral oil, 90, 98, 155
Minerals (trace elements), 3, 179, 187–90 (*see also* specific kinds); chelated, 8, 9, 171; in juices, 195–96; vitamins and (*see* Vitamins)
Moisturizer, skin, 99
Moore, Mary Tyler, 3, 95, 97
Mouth: drooping, makeup for, 114; exercises for, 59, 62; and teeth cleanliness, 157–58; and voice (*see* Voice); wash for, 158
Mugwort, 174; bath, 153–54, 155
Muscles, exercises for. *See* Exercises; specific body parts, kinds, problems

Nails. *See* Fingernails; Toenails
Naturopathy, 3, 44
Neck (neck muscles), exercises for, 57, 129–32
Nettle, 174
Niacin. *See under* B (B complex) vitamins
Nicotine. *See* Smoking
Night blindness, 90
Northen, Dr. Charles, 188
Nose, makeup for problem areas, 107–8
Nucleic acid, use of, 181–82
Nucleic Acid Therapy in Aging and Degenerative Disease (Frank), 181
Nutradyn, 65
Nutrition. *See* Food
Nuts, 42, 43

Oatmeal: bath, 155; soap, 154; and sunburn, 54, 55
Odor: body, 155–56; deodorants, 155–56; fragrance (perfumes), 153, 157; mouth, 158; tobacco, 7
Oil bath, 155
Oily hair, 72; conditioners for, 73; herbal rinse for, 78
Oily skin: cleansers, 48; facials, 52; makeup for, 99
Onion leaves, 174–75
Overweight (obesity), 38, 40, 125–27; corrective exercises, 127–45; dieting and, 125–26 (*see also* Dieting); fasting and, 7; plastic surgery and, 149–51; starches and sugars and, 38, 40; thyroid problem and exercise for, 145

P, vitamin, 187
Paba (para-aminobenzoic acid), 184–85; as a sun block, 53, 80
Pantothenic acid (panthenol), 76, 161, 184
Pants. *See* Slacks (pants)
Papaya leaves (papain), 175
Parks, Betty Garrett, 84
Parton, Dolly, 82
Peach leaves, 175
Peels and lifts, face. *See under* Face
Pencil: eye, 95, 98, 99, 115; lip, 105, 114
Perfumes (fragrance), 153, 157
Perspiration (*see also* Odor): bathing and, 153ff.; deodorants, 155–56; facial, makeup for, 123
Petroleum (petrolatum), 48, 98
Phosphorus, 188, 196
Photography: clothes and, 124; hair in, 83–84; makeup for, 123–24
Pill, the, 9, 45–46, 65–66, 183
Plastic surgery (cosmetic surgery), 66–69, 149–51; bust, 149–51; eyes, 93–94; face, 66–69; flab on upper arms, 135; hip pinch, 151; tummy tuck, 151
Plucking eyebrows. *See* Tweezing (plucking) eyebrows
Pollution, air, skin care and, 47
Posture, 145–47; sitting, 147; walking, 146–47
Potassium, 126, 188, 195, 196
Potato(es), 43; compress for eyes, 91
Powder: blush, 99; face, 99, 103, 123; puffs, use of, 98, 123

INDEX

Premarin, 9
Progesterone deficiency, 66
Protein, 3, 37, 38–40, 43, 126–27, 179 (*see also* specific foods, kinds); and food combinations, 199, 200; for hair, 71, 75; liquid diet, avoiding, 126; meal-planning guide and calories and, 191, 197–98; need for, sources of, and calories in, 38–40, 191–99
Provitamin, 175
Psoriasis, 45, 64
Puffiness, eye, 90, 91
Pumice stone, use of, 162
Pyridoxine. *See under* B (B complex) vitamins

Quassia bark, 175

Rashes, herbs for, 169
Red hair rinses, 81–82
Rejuvenating facial mask, 50
Riboflavin. *See under* B (B complex) vitamins
Rinse, Dr. Jacobus, and formula for a healthy heart, 41–42, 49
Rinses, finishing (hair). *See* Finishing rinses
RNA and DNA, 8, 44, 181, 182
Rosebuds, 175
Rose hips, 187
Rosemary, 154, 175–76; hair rinse, 77
Rouges, use of, 99; color chart, 104
Roughage. *See* Fiber
Rutin, 187

Saffiotti, Dr. Umberto, 181
Salads and dressings, 42. *See also* Vegetables
Salicylic acid. *See* Aspirin
Salt, use of (*see also* Sodium): and eye puffiness, 90
Scalp (*see also* Hair): massage of, 72, 74
Seafood (*see also* Fish): protein and calories and, 197–98
Seventh Day Adventists, 39
Shampooing (shampoos), 71–72, 73–75; beer, 75; combing wet hair and, 74; dry, 75; drying hair, 74; egg, 75; finishing rinses, 74, 76–78, 79, 81 (*see also* Finishing rinses); kinds to use, 75; pre-shampoo, 72–73; water temperature for, 73

Shaving (legs, under arms), 156–57
Shoulder problems, clothes and, 149
Shoulder stand, 25, 62
Showers (showering), 6–7, 15, 153–55. *See also* Cleanliness
Shute, Dr. Wilfred, 9
Silicone bust implants, 150–51
Sitting, posture and, 147
Sit-ups, 21–22, 145
Skin (skin care and problems), 37–69 (*see also* Face); acne, 64–66, 181; avoiding drugs and, 44–45; checking, 46; cleanliness and, 47–48, 153–58 (*see also* Cleanliness); cleansers, 47–48; diet and, 41–43; dry, 48; exercises for the face and, 55–63; facials, 48, 49–52, 54 (*see also* Facials); fasting and, 6–7; herbs for, 169–77 *passim;* makeup and, 97–123 (*see also* Makeup); moisturizer, 99; oily, 48; plastic surgery and, 66–69 (*see also* Plastic surgery); sunlight and, 53–55; tightener, 50; vitamins and, 180, 181–82, 185; zinc and, 43–44
Skin color, makeup color chart for, 104–5
Skin shake, 49, 161
Slacks (pants), heavy hips and, 149
Smoking, 7–8; tobacco breath and odor, 7; vitamin C and, 90
Soaps (detergents), 48; bath (oatmeal), 154; and hands, 160
Sodium, 188, 195, 196. *See also* Salt
Southernwood, 176
Sprouts, 39, 42
Stanwyck, Barbara, 147
Starches and sugars, 38, 40, 199, 200, 201. *See also* Carbohydrates; Sugar; specific kinds
Stomach (stomach muscles): exercises for, 21–22, 23–24, 29, 133–34, 145; tighteners, corrective exercises and, 133–34, 145; tummy tuck (plastic surgery), 151
Streisand, Barbra, 1, 93, 162
Stretch and pull exercises, 11–14
Sugar (*see also* Honey): refined, 38, 40; and starches (*see* Starches and sugars); and syrups, 201
Sunlight (sunburn): eyes and, 92; hair care and, 80; herbs for, 172, 173; lotions and, 53; makeup and, 97–98; skin care and, 53–55; sunburn treatment and, 53–55

Support hose, use of, 163
Surgery, cosmetic. *See* Plastic surgery
Swimming, chlorine in water and hair care, 80

Tannin, 77, 174, 176; tea bags for eyes, 91
Teeth (tooth care), cleanliness and, 157–58; mouthwash, 158; toothpaste, 158
Theobromine, 176
Thiamine. *See under* B (B complex) vitamins
Thighs (*see also* Hips): exercises for, 19–20, 30–35, 142–44; plastic surgery and, 151
Thyroid (thyroid problems): exercises for, 25, 145; and fingernails, 161; and overweight, exercise for, 145; zinc and, 190
Tiegs, Cheryl, 86
Tightener, skin, 50
Tobacco. *See* Smoking
Toenails, 163–64; cutting, 164
Torso and waist exercises. *See* Waist and torso exercises
Toxins (poisons): acne and, 64, 181; aspirin and, 45; bathing and, 154; eye appearance and, 90; fasting and, 6–7; feet and, 154, 162; in food, 5, 6; zinc as an antitoxin, 190
Trace elements. *See* Minerals; specific kinds, uses
Turkey. *See* Fowl
Tweezing (plucking) eyebrows, 94, 118, 119, 120, 121; how to, 121

Valerian (herb), 155, 176
Vapor baths, 154
Vaseline, use of, 98
Vegetable oils. *See* Fats (oils), dietary
Vegetables, 40, 191–93; and food combinations, 200; juices, 195–96; meal-planning guide and calories and, 191–93; non-starchy and green, 202; salads

Vegetables (*Continued*)
and dressings, 42; vitamins and minerals in, 179, 180, 195–96
Vertical scissors (exercise), 30–31
Vinegar, cider, for sunburn, 54
Vitamins, 3, 8–9, 179–87 (*see also* A, vitamin; B [B complex] vitamins; C, vitamin; D, vitamin; E, vitamin; P, vitamin); and acne, 65–66; and eyes, 90; fat-soluble and water-soluble, 179; in juices, 195–96; kinds, need for, and food sources of, 179–87 (*see also* specific foods, vitamins); minerals and, 179, 187–90; and plastic surgery, 69; what to take, 69
Voice (diction, enunciation, language), 165–68; care of, 167; diaphragm breathing and, 167; exercises for, 166, 168; glottic shock and, 167; laughing and, 167; timbre and, 166; tone and, 166; vocal cords and, 166

Waist and torso exercises, 14, 16, 17–18, 133–34; corrective, 133–34
Walk(ing), posture and, 146–47
Wardrobe. *See* Clothes
Warts, celandine for, 170–71
Water, drinking, 6, 8, 9
Weight problem. *See* Overweight; specific problems
Wheat germ, use of, 42, 182, 183
Whiteheads, 64
Wigs, 82–83
Wild cherry, 176
Willow bark, 177
Wrinkles, 47, 63; eyes, 90; frown lines, 55, 56; vitamins and, 181

Yarrow, 177
Yellow dock, 177
Yoghurt, 41, 42, 43. *See also* Kefir

Zinc, 43–44; need for and food sources of, 190